Dear Reader,

How do you feel when you wake up in the morning? Are you refreshed and ready to go, or groggy and grumpy? For many people, the second scenario is all too common. More than one in three adults get less than the recommended seven or more hours of sleep each night, according to the Centers for Disease Control and Prevention. Insomnia—trouble falling or staying asleep—is the most common complaint. But other chronic disorders, including sleep apnea, restless legs syndrome, or narcolepsy, can also contribute to a shut-eye shortfall. Sometimes, unavoidable stress or problems like a death in the family keep you up at night. But so can habits that you can control, such as drinking alcohol or caffeine at night or using brightly lit electronic devices too close to bedtime.

Whatever the cause, the toll of all that lost sleep on health, well-being, and productivity is enormous. Insufficient sleep can make you too tired to work efficiently, to exercise, or to eat healthfully. Over time, sleep deprivation increases the risk for a number of chronic health problems, including obesity, diabetes, high blood pressure, and heart disease. What's more, according to a government report, one in 25 American drivers admitted to falling asleep while driving at least once in the previous month. Some estimates suggest drowsy driving accounts for up to a quarter of fatal highway crashes. And according to a 2017 report from the Rand Corporation, the United States loses an equivalent of 1.2 million working days because of insufficient sleep, which translates to economic losses of up to $411 billion each year.

Fortunately, you needn't fumble about in a fog of fatigue. This report features the latest information on sleep problems, ranging from insomnia to sleep-related eating disorder, and it details the various treatments available. Sleep medications are not necessarily the best option. Growing evidence backs the use of cognitive behavioral therapy, a drug-free approach to treating insomnia, which is now available not only through clinicians, but also via websites and smartphone apps. You'll learn about the many devices and procedures that are available for treating sleep apnea, as well as related techniques that can reduce snoring. You'll learn tips and tricks for coping with jet lag and how to get back on a normal schedule if you're a night owl. Other problems covered here include narcolepsy and restless legs syndrome. Whatever your sleep issue, you'll learn about reliable, time-tested remedies to help you get the sleep you need for optimal health, safety, and well-being.

Sincerely,

*Lawrence Epstein*

Lawrence Epstein, M.D.
*Medical Editor*

# Sleep mechanics

For centuries, scientists scrutinized minute aspects of human activity, but showed little interest in the time that people spent in sleep. Sleep seemed inaccessible to medical probing—a subject best suited to poets and dream interpreters who could conjure meaning out of the void. It was thought to be no more than a natural response to the darkness and silence of night, when the brain could no longer react to the sensory stimulation of the day. As a result, scientists believed the brain simply "turned off" and remained unchanged throughout the night.

All that changed in the 1930s, when researchers found they could place sensitive electrodes on the scalp and record the signals produced by electrical activity in the brain to create electroencephalograms, or EEGs. When this technique revealed lively brain activity even in sleeping subjects, scientists realized that sleep did not represent a void, but was in fact a dynamic time, incorporating different stages with markedly different patterns of brain waves. Further study revealed that it is a period when the brain encodes new memories or information that it wants to keep (a process called consolidation), when it cleans out toxins, when growth and development occur, and when the immune system surveys the body for potential problems.

Far from being a luxury, sleep is now known to be essential, required for health and optimal functioning. In fact, sleep deprivation can be used as a form of torture. Yet many of us continue to get inadequate sleep—either because we deliberately deprive ourselves of sleep or because we seem unable to get a good night's rest.

This report will delve into the many steps you can take to restore sleep quality. But first, it may help to examine the different stages of sleep and what scientists call "sleep architecture," meaning the patterns of alternating sleep stages you pass through during the night.

Scientists used to think that sleep served no purpose, but was simply a response to the darkness at night. Now they know that sleep is essential to a person's health and well-being.

## Quiet (non-REM) sleep

Scientists divide sleep into two major types: REM (rapid eye movement) sleep or dreaming sleep, and non-REM sleep, also known as quiet sleep. Surprisingly, they are as different from each other as either one is from waking.

Sleep specialists have called non-REM sleep "an idling brain in a movable body." During this phase, thinking and most bodily functions slow down, but movement can still occur, and a person often shifts position while sinking into deeper stages of sleep.

To an extent, the idea of "dropping" into sleep parallels changes in brain-wave patterns at the onset of non-REM sleep. When you are awake, billions of brain cells receive and analyze sensory information and coordinate behavior by sending electrical impulses to one another. If you're fully awake, an EEG records a messy, irregular scribble of activity. Once your eyes are closed and your brain no longer receives visual input, brain waves settle into a steady and rhythmic pattern of about 10 cycles per second. This is the alpha-wave pattern, characteristic of calm, relaxed wakefulness (see Figure 1, page 3).

The transition to quiet sleep is a quick one that might be likened to flipping a switch—that is, you are either awake (switch on) or asleep (switch off). Some brain centers and pathways stimulate the entire brain to wakefulness; others promote falling asleep. One brain chemical, hypocretin (also called orexin), seems to play an important role in regulating when the flip between states occurs and keeping you in the new state. Interestingly, people with a condition called narcolepsy often lack hypocretin, and as a result they frequently flip back and forth between sleep and wakefulness, suddenly falling asleep during the day or at other inappropriate times for short bouts known as "sleep attacks."

Unless something disturbs the process, you proceed smoothly through the three stages of quiet sleep.

## Stage N1

In making the transition from wakefulness into light sleep, you spend about five minutes in stage N1 sleep. On the EEG, the predominant brain waves slow to four to seven cycles per second, a pattern called theta waves (see Figure 1, at right). Body temperature begins to drop, muscles relax, and eyes often move slowly from side to side. People in stage N1 sleep lose awareness of their surroundings, but they are easily jarred awake. However, not everyone experiences stage N1 sleep in the same way: if awakened, one person might recall being drowsy, while another might describe having been asleep.

## Stage N2 (light sleep)

This first stage of true sleep lasts 10 to 25 minutes. Your eyes are still, and your heart rate and breathing are slower than when awake. Your brain's electrical activity is irregular. EEG tracings record two patterns that occur almost exclusively in this stage of sleep:

- Sleep spindles are brief bursts of activity in which brain waves speed up for roughly half a second or longer between larger, slower waves. Scientists believe that when spindles occur, the brain disconnects from outside sensory input and begins the process of memory consolidation (which involves organizing memories for long-term storage).
- K-complexes are some of the largest waves seen on

an EEG. Scientists think they represent a sort of built-in vigilance system that keeps you poised to awaken if necessary. K-complexes can also be provoked by certain sounds or other external or internal stimuli. Whisper someone's name during stage N2 sleep, and a K-complex will appear on the EEG. You spend about half the night in stage N2 sleep.

## Stage N3 (deep sleep, or slow-wave sleep)

Eventually, large, slow brain waves called delta waves become a major feature on the EEG, and you enter deep sleep. Breathing becomes more regular. Blood pressure falls, and the pulse slows to about 20% to

## Figure 1: EEG brain-wave patterns during sleep

Brain waves change dramatically during the different stages of sleep.

30% below the waking rate. The brain is less responsive to external stimuli, making it difficult to wake the sleeper.

Deep sleep seems to be a time for your body to renew and repair itself. Blood flow is directed less toward your brain, which cools measurably. At the beginning of this stage, the pituitary gland releases a pulse of growth hormone that stimulates tissue growth and muscle repair. Researchers have also detected increased blood levels of substances that activate your immune system, raising the possibility that deep sleep helps the body defend itself against infection.

Normally, young people spend about 20% of their sleep time in stretches of deep sleep lasting up to half an hour, but deep sleep is vastly reduced in most people over age 65 (see "The later years," page 9). When you sleep after a period of sleep deprivation, you pass quickly through the lighter sleep stages into the deeper stages and spend a greater proportion of sleep time there. This suggests that deep sleep plays a large part in restoring alertness and fills an essential role in a person's optimal functioning.

## Dreaming (REM) sleep

Dreaming occurs during REM sleep, which has been described as "an active brain in a paralyzed body." Your brain races, thinking and dreaming, as your eyes dart back and forth rapidly behind closed lids. Your body temperature rises. Your blood pressure increases, and your heart rate and breathing speed up to daytime levels. The sympathetic nervous system, which

### Why do we dream?

Many people are fascinated by dreams and wonder if the seemingly random thoughts, images, and sensations that occur during sleep hold any special meaning or purpose. Certain themes or scenarios in dreams may be common across time and cultures, according to an article in *Psychology Today*. An example is discovering a new room or passage in your home, which leads to a magical place. Another classic dream is realizing that you are about to debut in a play or take an important test or deliver a major project at work, but you've done nothing to prepare for it and can't possibly fake your way through it. Other common themes include being chased or pursued, falling, flying, and having sexual experiences.

Although many explanations have been offered, the meaning and function of dreams is still a matter of debate. Following are some of the competing theories.

**Hidden desires.** One famous work on the subject, Sigmund Freud's *The Interpretation of Dreams*, published in 1899, explored why people dream and what dreams reveal about their psychological lives. Freud believed that dreams reveal hidden conflicts, desires, and fears, albeit in disguised form. Other psychoanalytic thinkers later elaborated on and refined his ideas, suggesting that dreams help people organize their thoughts as well as consolidate and reinforce their long-term memories.

**Random impulses.** The technological advances that enabled EEG recordings during sleep gave rise to alternate theories, like the "activation synthesis hypothesis," which holds that dreams are triggered by random electrical impulses generated during REM sleep. The dream is the brain's attempt to make sense and a cohesive story out of the randomly generated memories. In this theory, the meaning of the dreams is not significant, and the evidence is that we remember so few of them. (In fact, whether or not you can remember a dream seems to depend mainly on one factor—how close to the dreaming period you wake up. However, people can train themselves to remember dreams better by writing them down when they wake up.)

**Threat simulation.** In yet another interpretation, evolutionary psychologists point to the well-documented realistic aspects of dreams as evidence that dreams serve a purpose. The "threat simulation theory" suggests that dreams in which people react to a threatening event help them rehearse for danger in real life. This mental practice during sleep, they postulate, may have offered a survival advantage.

**Learning and memory.** Several lines of evidence point to the importance of dreaming for learning and memory. For example, newborns and young children, who are in a period of intense learning, spend far more time in REM sleep than adults. According to Dr. Robert Stickgold and colleagues at Harvard's Beth Israel Deaconess Medical Center, dreams may help you process and learn from experiences during the day—perhaps enhancing your ability to remember them. However, REM is not solely responsible for memory consolidation. Both REM and non-REM sleep appear to play a role, with each enhancing different types of learning and memory.

While scientists continue to debate the precise purpose of dreaming, the fact that other species such as dogs dream, too, suggests that it plays a fundamental biological role. Life would certainly be less interesting without it.

creates the fight-or-flight response, is twice as active as when you're awake. Despite all this activity, your body hardly moves, except for intermittent twitches; muscles not needed for breathing or eye movement are quiet.

Just as deep sleep restores your body, scientists believe that REM or dreaming sleep restores your mind, perhaps in part by helping clear out irrelevant information. Studies of students' ability to solve a complex puzzle involving abstract shapes suggest the brain processes information overnight; students who got a good night's sleep after seeing the puzzle fared much better than those asked to solve the puzzle immediately. Earlier studies found that REM sleep facilitates learning and memory. People tested to measure how well they had learned a new task involving visual discrimination improved their scores after a night's sleep. If they were subjected to periodic awakenings that prevented them from having REM sleep, the improvements were lost. By contrast, if they were awakened an equal number of times from deep sleep, the improvements in the scores were unaffected. These findings may help explain why students who stay up all night cramming for an examination generally retain less information than classmates who get some sleep.

About three to five times a night, or about every 90 minutes, you enter REM sleep. The first such episode usually lasts for only a few minutes, but REM time increases progressively over the course of the night. The final period of REM sleep may last a half-hour. If you're deprived of REM sleep and then allowed a subsequent night of undisturbed sleep, you will enter this stage earlier and spend a higher proportion of sleep time in it—a phenomenon called REM rebound.

## Sleep architecture

During the night, a normal sleeper moves between different sleep stages in a fairly predictable pattern, alternating between REM and non-REM sleep. When these stages are charted on a diagram, called a hypnogram (see Figure 2, above right), the different levels resemble a drawing of a city skyline. Sleep experts call this pattern sleep architecture.

In a young adult, normal sleep architecture usually

### Figure 2: Sleep architecture

When experts chart sleep stages on a hypnogram, the different levels resemble a drawing of a city skyline. This pattern is known as sleep architecture. The hypnogram above shows a typical night's sleep of a healthy young adult.

consists of four or five alternating non-REM and REM periods. Most deep sleep occurs in the first half of the night. As the night progresses, periods of REM sleep get longer and alternate with stage N2 sleep. Later in life, the sleep skyline will change, with less stage N3 sleep, more stage N1 sleep, and more awakenings.

Control of many of the features of sleep architecture resides in the brainstem, the area that also controls breathing, blood pressure, and heartbeat. Fluctuating activity in the nerve cells and the chemical messengers they produce seem to coordinate the timing of wakefulness, arousal, and the periodic changeover that occurs several times a night between REM and non-REM sleep.

Several neurotransmitters (brain chemicals that neurons release to communicate with adjacent cells) play a role in arousal. Adenosine and gamma-aminobutyric acid (GABA) are believed to promote sleep. Acetylcholine regulates REM sleep. Norepinephrine, epinephrine, dopamine, and hypocretin stimulate wakefulness. Individuals vary greatly in their natural levels of neurotransmitters and in their sensitivity to these chemicals. Many sleep medications are designed to mimic or counteract their effects.

## Your internal clock

Certain brain structures and chemicals produce the states of sleeping and waking. For instance, a pacemaker-like mechanism in the brain regulates circa-

## Figure 3: The sleep/wake control center

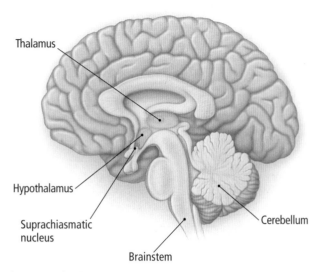

The pacemaker-like mechanism in your brain that regulates the circadian rhythm of sleeping and waking is thought to be located in the suprachiasmatic nucleus. This cluster of cells is part of the hypothalamus, the brain center that regulates appetite, body temperature, and other biological states.

dian rhythms. ("Circadian" means "about a day.") This internal clock, which gradually becomes established during the first months of life, controls the daily ups and downs of biological patterns, including body temperature, blood pressure, and the release of hormones.

Circadian rhythms make people's desire for sleep strongest between midnight and dawn, and to a lesser extent in midafternoon. In one study, researchers instructed a group of people to try to stay awake for 24 hours. Not surprisingly, many slipped into naps despite their best efforts not to. When the investigators plotted the times when these unplanned naps occurred, they found peaks between 2 a.m. and 4 a.m. and between 2 p.m. and 3 p.m.

Most Americans sleep during the night as dictated by their circadian rhythms, although many who work on weekdays nap in the afternoon on the weekends. In societies where taking a siesta is the norm, people can respond to their bodies' daily dips in alertness with a one- to two-hour afternoon nap during the workday and a correspondingly shorter sleep at night.

In the 1970s, studies in rats identified a brain structure called the suprachiasmatic nucleus as the location of the internal clock. This cluster of cells is part of the hypothalamus, the brain center that regulates appetite and other biological states (see Figure 3, at left). When this tiny area was damaged, the sleep/wake rhythm disappeared and the rats no longer slept on a normal schedule. Although the clock is largely self-regulating, its location allows it to respond to several types of external cues to keep it set at 24 hours. Scientists call these cues "zeitgebers," a German word meaning "time givers." They include the following:

**Light.** Light striking your eyes is the most influential zeitgeber. When researchers invited volunteers into the laboratory and exposed them to light at intervals that were at odds with the outside world, the participants unconsciously reset their biological clocks to match the new light input. Exposure to light at the right time helps keep the circadian clock on the correct time schedule. However, exposure at the wrong time can shift sleep and wakefulness to undesired times. The circadian rhythm disturbances and sleep problems that affect up to 90% of blind people demonstrate the importance of light to sleep/wake patterns.

**Time.** As a person reads clocks, follows work and train schedules, and demands that the body remain alert for certain tasks and social events, there is cognitive pressure to stay on schedule.

**Melatonin.** Cells in the suprachiasmatic nucleus contain receptors for melatonin, a hormone produced in a predictable daily rhythm by the pineal gland, which is located deep in the brain between the two hemispheres. Levels of melatonin begin climbing after dark and ebb after dawn. The hormone induces drowsiness, and scientists believe its daily light-sensitive cycles help keep the sleep/wake cycle on track. ▼

# Sleep changes throughout life

To a certain extent, heredity determines how people sleep throughout their lives. Identical twins, for example, have much more similar sleep patterns than nonidentical twins or other sibling pairs. Scientists have also discovered two genetic mutations relating to sleep duration (see "A gene that affects circadian rhythms," below right). However, many factors can affect how a person sleeps. Aging is the most important influence on basic sleep rhythms—from age 20 on, it takes progressively longer to fall asleep. You sleep less each night, stages N1 and N2 sleep increase, deep sleep and REM decrease, and you awaken more often during the night (see Table 1, page 8).

## Childhood

For an adult to sleep like a baby is not only unrealistic but also undesirable. A newborn may sleep eight times a day, accumulating 17 hours of sleep and spending about half of it in REM sleep (see Table 2, page 8). REM periods occur often, usually less than an hour apart.

At about the age of 4 weeks, a newborn's sleep periods get longer. By 6 months, infants spend longer

A newborn may sleep 17 hours a day, spending about half of it in REM sleep (dreaming sleep). By 6 months, infants begin sleeping through the night and spend more time in non-REM sleep.

and more regular periods in non-REM sleep; most begin sleeping through the night and taking naps in the morning and afternoon. During the preschool years, daytime naps gradually shorten, until by age 6 most children are awake all day and sleep for about 10 hours a night.

Between age 7 and puberty, nocturnal melatonin production is at its lifetime peak, and sleep at this age is deep and restorative. At this age, if a child is sleepy during the day, parents should be concerned.

### A gene that affects circadian rhythms

Whether you're a night owl or an early riser, you probably know roughly how long you need to sleep to feel fully rested. Some people feel perky after just seven hours of sleep, while others are groggy if they log less than nine hours. The discovery of genetic mutations in people who need far less sleep than average helps explain at least some of this variation. Scientists discovered two such mutations in a gene called DEC2, which is known to affect circadian rhythms.

The first mutation was found in a mother and daughter who were naturally short sleepers, requiring just six hours a night instead of the average of eight. Many Americans sleep just six hours nightly, but most rely on alarms, caffeine, and power naps to awaken and stay awake during the day. By contrast, these two women awoke naturally after six hours. The scientists then created genetically engineered mice with the same mutation. The mice not only slept less and stayed awake longer, they also needed less sleep to recover following sleep deprivation.

The same researchers later discovered a different DEC2 mutation in a pair of fraternal twins, one with the mutation and one without. The twin with the mutation slept, on average, two hours less than his twin and needed far less time to recover from sleep deprivation.

Now, an international team is sequencing other so-called CLOCK genes, which are involved in regulating circadian rhythms. The findings may help scientists better understand the nature of sleep and perhaps pave the way for new drugs to treat sleep disorders.

## Table 1: Sleep changes during adulthood

As people age, it takes longer to fall asleep, a phenomenon called increased sleep latency. And sleep efficiency—the percentage of time spent asleep while in bed—decreases as well.

| | AGE 20 | AGE 40 | AGE 60 | AGE 70 | AGE 80 |
|---|---|---|---|---|---|
| Time to fall asleep | 16 minutes | 17 minutes | 18 minutes | 18.5 minutes | 19 minutes |
| Total sleep time | 7.5 hours | 7 hours | 6.2 hours | 6 hours | 5.8 hours |
| Time in stage N2 sleep | 47% | 51% | 53% | 55% | 57% |
| Time in stage N3 sleep | 20% | 15% | 10% | 9% | 7.5% |
| Time in REM sleep | 22% | 21% | 20% | 19% | 17% |
| Time asleep while in bed | 95% | 88% | 84% | 82% | 79% |

Source: Sleep, Nov. 1, 2004, pp. 1255–73.

## Table 2: Sleep needs throughout life

The amount of sleep you need each day changes as you grow older.

| AGE GROUP | | RECOMMENDED HOURS OF SLEEP PER DAY |
|---|---|---|
| Newborn | 0–3 months | 14–17 hours |
| Infant | 4–12 months | 12–16 hours per 24 hours (including naps) |
| Toddler | 1–2 years | 11–14 hours per 24 hours (including naps) |
| Preschool | 3–5 years | 10–13 hours per 24 hours (including naps) |
| School age | 6–12 years | 9–12 hours per 24 hours |
| Teen | 13–18 years | 8–10 hours per 24 hours |
| Adult | 18–60 years | 7 or more hours per night |
| | 61–64 years | 7–9 hours |
| | 65 years and older | 7–8 hours |

Source: CDC.

## Adolescence

Teenagers still need about eight to 10 hours of sleep each night. But starting around adolescence, most of them sleep less than they need. Many factors contribute to the problem, such as drinking caffeinated beverages or staying up too late doing homework or texting friends. But teens' natural sleep/wake cycles also begin to shift up to two hours later once they reach puberty. That means they may not be sleepy until well after their bedtime the night before and may have difficulty waking up early enough to get to school on time.

Research shows that early high school start times contribute to sleep deprivation among teens, which can lead to mood swings, behavioral problems, and difficulties with concentration and learning. Adolescents who get enough sleep are less likely to be overweight, suffer from depression, or be involved in a car accident. They're also more likely to have better grades and a higher quality of life. In response to this evidence, the American Academy of Pediatrics has issued a policy statement recommending that middle and high schools delay start times to 8:30 a.m. or later.

## Adulthood

During young adulthood, sleep patterns usually seem stable but in fact are slowly evolving. Between age 20 and age 30, the amount of deep sleep drops by about half, and nighttime awakenings double. By age 40, deep sleep is markedly reduced.

Women's reproductive cycles can greatly influence sleep. During the first trimester of pregnancy, many women are sleepy all the time and may log an extra two hours a night if their schedules permit. As pregnancy continues, hormonal and anatomical changes make sound, restful sleeping a challenge, so less of a woman's time in bed is actually spent sleeping. As a result, fatigue increases (see "Getting a good night's sleep during pregnancy," page 9). After giving birth, women are often exhausted. Not only are they at the mercy of their newborn's erratic sleep schedule, but breastfeeding also promotes sleepiness. Some research suggests that sleep disturbances during and after pregnancy may contribute to postpartum depression.

Women who aren't pregnant may notice that their sleep habits shift throughout the month. During the second half of the menstrual cycle, progesterone levels rise, which tends to make women more drowsy than

## Getting a good night's sleep during pregnancy

In a National Sleep Foundation poll, nearly eight in 10 women reported disturbed sleep during pregnancy. Here are some tips to help you get a better night's sleep when you're expecting:

✔ Avoid spicy, fried, or acidic foods (such as tomato products), which contribute to heartburn.

✔ If you have heartburn, raise the head of your bed by placing blocks under the bed's legs.

✔ Prevent nausea by eating frequent snacks during the day.

✔ If you feel drowsy, take a midday nap for up to 30 minutes, which can help you feel more refreshed but won't interfere with nighttime sleep.

✔ Exercise regularly to reduce leg cramps and improve sleep.

✔ Cut down on fluids before bedtime to reduce nighttime trips to the bathroom.

✔ Use pillows or special pregnancy cushions to support your abdomen.

when levels are lower during the first half of the cycle. When both progesterone and estrogen levels fall a few days prior to menstruation, many women have trouble sleeping—one of the main symptoms of premenstrual syndrome, or PMS.

**Snooze news** | The average length of time Americans spend sleeping has dropped from about nine hours a night in 1910 to about seven hours today.

## Middle age

As men and women enter middle age, deep sleep continues to diminish. Nighttime awakenings become more frequent and last longer. Waking after about three hours of sleep is particularly common. During menopause, many women experience hot flashes that can interrupt sleep. Obese people are more prone to nocturnal breathing problems, which often start during middle age. Men and women who are physically fit sleep more soundly as they grow older, compared with their sedentary peers.

## The later years

In older adults, REM sleep decreases a small amount, but still hovers around 20% of total sleep time. Other changes are more pronounced. Deep sleep accounts for less than 10% of sleep time, and in some people it is completely absent. Falling asleep takes longer,

and the shallow quality of sleep results in dozens of awakenings during the night. Doctors used to reassure older people that they needed less sleep than younger ones to function well, but sleep experts now know that isn't true. At any age, most adults need seven or more hours of sleep to function at their best. Because of the frequent fragmentation of sleep, it can take longer in bed to get the same amount of sleep. If older people are unable to get all the required sleep at night, they often supplement nighttime sleep with daytime naps. This can be a successful strategy for accumulating sufficient total sleep over a 24-hour period. However, if you find that you need a nap, it's best to take one midday nap, rather than several brief ones scattered throughout the day and evening.

Sleep disturbances in elderly people, particularly in those who have Alzheimer's disease or other forms of dementia, are very disruptive for the individuals they affect and their caregivers. In one study, 70% of caregivers cited these problems as the decisive factor in seeking nursing home placement for a loved one. ▼

# Dangers of sleep deprivation

Lack of sufficient sleep can lead to a range of ill effects, triggering mild to potentially life-threatening consequences, from weight gain to a heart attack (see Figure 4, below). Sleep deprivation is broadly categorized as complete or partial, based on duration and severity. Complete sleep deprivation happens when you pull an all-nighter. Partial sleep deprivation happens when you stint on sleep for a number of nights in a row (for example, only getting six hours of sleep each night for two weeks). But the mental and physical effects are similar.

## Complete sleep deprivation

Normally, you're up for 16 or 17 hours before going to bed. As waking hours extend beyond this point, you first feel tired, then exhausted. Simple tasks that you would normally have no trouble accomplishing start to become difficult. In fact, a number of studies of hand-eye coordination and reaction time have shown that such sleep deprivation can be as debilitating as intoxication.

In one study, volunteers stayed awake for 28 hours (from 8 a.m. to noon the following day) and took tests of hand-eye coordination every 30 minutes during that time. On another day, the same volunteers completed the tests after drinking 10 to 15 grams of alcohol at 30-minute intervals until their blood alcohol content reached 0.10%—enough to be charged with driving while intoxicated in most states. The study concluded that 24 hours of wakefulness caused as much impairment as a blood alcohol content of 0.10%.

Sleep deprivation also leaves you prone to dozing off at the wheel and losing your concentration—two potentially dangerous phenomena that play a role in thousands of transportation accidents each year (see "Microsleeps and automatic behavior," page 11). When people don't sleep at all for two to three days, they have difficulty completing tasks that demand a high attention level and often experience mood swings, depression, and increased feelings of tension. Sleep deprivation is so debilitating that it is sometimes used as a component of military interrogation.

Performance is also highly influenced by fluctuations in circadian rhythms. For example, sleep-deprived people may still function fairly well during the morning and evening. But during the peaks of sleepiness in the afternoon and overnight hours, people often literally cannot stay awake and may fall asleep while standing, sitting, or even while talking on the telephone, working on the computer, or eating. A small percentage experience paranoia and hallucinations.

---

## Figure 4: Health consequences of insufficient sleep

People who skimp on sleep face a higher risk of numerous health problems.

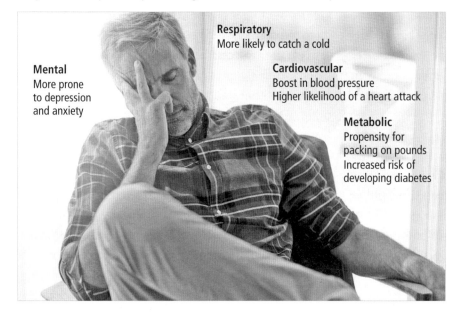

**Mental**
More prone to depression and anxiety

**Respiratory**
More likely to catch a cold

**Cardiovascular**
Boost in blood pressure
Higher likelihood of a heart attack

**Metabolic**
Propensity for packing on pounds
Increased risk of developing diabetes

© Jeffhtergen | Getty Images

### ▶ Microsleeps and automatic behavior

Microsleeps are brief episodes of sleep that occur in the midst of ongoing wakeful activity. They can happen in people who are sleep deprived, often without their awareness. These are the head nods some people experience when trying to stay awake during a lecture, for example. They usually last just a few seconds but can go on for 10 or 15 seconds—and pose a grave danger if they happen when a person is driving. Brain-wave monitoring by EEG of someone experiencing microsleeps shows brief periods of stage N1 sleep intruding into wakefulness. During this time, the brain does not respond to noise or other sensory inputs, and you don't react to things happening around you. Because people are poor judges of when microsleeps will occur (and are equally poor at preventing them), they're a major factor in many motor vehicle accidents.

Automatic behavior refers to a period of several minutes or more during which a person is awake and performing routine duties but not attending to his or her surroundings or responding to changes in the environment. These episodes occur when people are extremely sleepy and are another consequence of sleep deprivation. Examples include a driver who keeps the car on the road but misses an intended exit and a train engineer who can continue pressing a lever at regular intervals but doesn't notice an obstruction on the track.

## Partial sleep deprivation

Partial sleep deprivation occurs when you get some sleep, but not 100% of what you need. Experts refer to this as building up a sleep debt.

After a single night of short sleep, most people function at or near their normal level. They may not feel great, but they can usually get through the day without others noticing that anything is amiss. After two or more nights of short sleep, people usually show signs of irritability and sleepiness. Work performance begins to suffer—particularly on complicated tasks— and people are more likely to complain of headaches, stomach problems, sore joints, memory lapses, and sluggish reaction time. In addition, people face a far higher risk of falling asleep on the job or while driving.

Long-term partial sleep deprivation occurs when someone gets less than the optimal amount of sleep for months or years on end—a common scenario for insomniacs and people with sleep disorders. But even healthy people may fall prey to this problem, if they can't resist the round-the-clock opportunities for commerce, communication, and entertainment that our 24/7 society now offers.

The health consequences may be serious. In a landmark study of human sleep deprivation, researchers followed a group of student volunteers who slept only four hours nightly for six consecutive days. The volunteers developed higher blood pressure and higher levels of the stress hormone cortisol, and they produced only half the usual number of antibodies to a flu vaccine. The sleep-deprived students also showed signs of insulin resistance—a condition that is the precursor of type 2 diabetes. All these changes—which were reversed when the students made up the hours of lost sleep—help explain why ongoing sleep debt raises the risk of a number of health problems. Also, note that, unlike the students in this study, most people don't manage to make up over the weekend for all the sleep they miss during the work week.

## How long-term sleep loss harms your health

A growing number of studies have linked long-term sleep deficits with significant health problems.

**Diabetes.** A report in *Diabetes Care* found a sharp increase in the risk of type 2 diabetes in people with persistent insomnia. People who had insomnia for a year or longer and who slept less than five hours per night had three times the risk of type 2 diabetes compared with those who had no sleep complaints and who slept six or more hours nightly. As with overweight and obesity (which are also closely linked to type 2 diabetes), the underlying cause is thought to involve a disruption of the body's normal hormonal regulation, but in this case, it results from insufficient sleep.

**High blood pressure.** Researchers involved in the diabetes study also evaluated risk of high blood pressure among the same group of people, which included more than 1,700 randomly chosen men and women from rural Pennsylvania. As described in the journal *Sleep*, the researchers found the risk of high blood pressure was three-and-a-half times greater among insomniacs who routinely slept less than six hours per night compared with normal sleepers who slept six or more hours nightly.

**Heart disease.** A number of studies have linked sleep deprivation with several well-known risk factors for heart disease, including higher cholesterol levels, higher triglyceride levels, and higher blood pressure. People who don't get sufficient sleep also have higher blood levels of stress hormones and substances that indicate inflammation, a key player in cardiovascular disease. Some research suggests that chronic sleep deprivation (getting no more than four hours a night) may double a woman's risk of dying of heart disease.

One common cause of poor sleep, sleep apnea (see page 31) also raises heart disease risk. The low oxygen and high carbon dioxide levels that occur in apnea-disturbed sleep raise levels of stress hormones. This boosts blood pressure and heart rate, putting stress on the cardiovascular system. Sleep apnea appears to increase the risk of heart attack, heart failure, and heart rhythm disorders such as atrial fibrillation. People with moderate to severe sleep apnea have three times the risk of stroke compared with people who don't have the condition.

In the Wisconsin Sleep Cohort study, people with severe sleep apnea were three times more likely to die of heart disease during 18 years of follow-up than those without apnea. When researchers excluded those who used a breathing machine (a common apnea treatment), the risk jumped to more than five times higher. Apnea spells can trigger arrhythmias (irregular heartbeats), and the condition also increases the risk of stroke and heart failure.

**Mental illness.** A study of about 1,000 adults ages 21 to 30 found that, compared with normal sleepers, those who reported a history of insomnia during an interview were four times as likely to develop major depression by the time of a second interview three years later. And two studies in young people—one involving 300 pairs of young twins, and another

including about 1,000 teenagers—found that sleep problems often developed before a diagnosis of major depression and (to a lesser extent) anxiety. Sleep problems in the teenagers preceded depression 69% of the time and anxiety disorders 27% of the time.

**Dementia.** A growing body of research suggests that sleep disturbances may increase the risk of developing Alzheimer's disease. A report that pooled findings from 27 observational studies found that people with sleep problems were nearly 1.7 times as likely to develop cognitive impairments or Alzheimer's than people without sleep issues. Experts believe that sleep helps clear the brain of amyloid, the protein thought to damage nerve cells in Alzheimer's. A 2018 study in *JAMA Neurology* found that older people with excessive daytime sleepiness were more likely to show increased amyloid in their brains over time. However, it's not yet clear whether disrupted sleep contributes to amyloid buildup or vice versa.

**Viral infections.** Anecdotal evidence supports the notion that when you're tired and run-down, you're more likely to get sick. A study in *Archives of Internal Medicine* offers some proof. Researchers tracked the sleep habits of 153 men and women for two weeks, then quarantined them for five days and exposed them to cold viruses. People who slept an average of less than seven hours per night were three times as likely to get sick as those who averaged at least eight hours.

**Weight gain.** Not getting enough sleep makes you more likely to gain weight, according to a review article in the journal *Obesity* that analyzed findings from 36 studies. The link appears to be especially strong among children. Lack of sufficient sleep tends to disrupt hormones that control hunger and appetite, causing you to eat hundreds of extra calories per day—in particular, quickly digested carbohydrates. What's more, the resulting daytime fatigue often discourages you from exercising. Excess weight, in turn, increases the risk of a number of health problems—including some of those listed above. ◗

# Practical tips for sounder sleep

Getting enough sleep is just as important as other vital elements of good health, such as eating a healthy diet, getting regular exercise, and practicing good dental hygiene. In short, sleep is not a luxury but a basic component of a healthy lifestyle. But just like purchasing healthy foods, taking an after-dinner walk, or flossing your teeth, getting adequate sleep requires time and discipline. Mentally block off certain hours for sleep and then follow through on your intention, avoid building up a sleep debt, and take steps to set up an ideal sleep environment. Seek a doctor's help if conventional steps toward good sleep, such as those in this chapter, don't work.

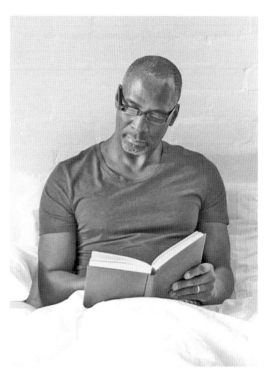

If you have trouble sleeping, avoid stimulating activities such as late-night exercise. Turn off devices after 9 p.m. (or two hours before bedtime). Try listening to soothing music or reading a book instead.

This doesn't mean that you can't have any fun, or that you need to get eight hours of sleep 365 days a year. Just as an occasional ice cream sundae won't make you fat, staying up a few extra hours for a party or to meet a deadline is perfectly acceptable—as long as you make plans to compensate the next day by taking a short afternoon nap or going to bed earlier. But over the long haul, you need to make sure you consistently get enough sleep.

Following are some ways to improve your sleep. These good habits are known as "sleep hygiene," because they represent scientific thinking about maintaining healthy sleep patterns.

## Create a sleep sanctuary

A sleep-friendly bedroom can make it easier to fall and stay asleep, so take time to address issues that affect what you hear, see, and feel while in bed.

**Control noise.** A quiet bedroom is especially important for older adults, who spend less time in deep sleep. As a result, they are more easily awakened by noises. Here are some ways to reduce or disguise noises that can interfere with sleep:

- Decorate with heavy curtains and rugs, which absorb sounds.
- Install double-paned windows.
- Use earplugs.
- Use a fan or a sleep machine, which provide "white noise," or a recording of soothing sounds, such as falling rain, croaking frogs, or chirping crickets.

**Dim bright light.** Bright light at night can suppress your body's

© Dean Mitchell | Getty Images

production of melatonin and make it harder to sleep. Keep your pre-bedtime light intake down with these steps:

- Avoid watching television or using a computer after 9 p.m.
- Don't read from a backlit electronic device (such as an iPad) at night. (Also see "Screening out blue light: Does it help?" below.)
- Replace bright lights with lower-wattage bulbs, or install dimmer switches that allow you to keep the lights low at night.

Bright bathroom lights can be an issue, especially since most people use the bathroom right before retiring (and often in the middle of the night). But you don't want to stumble if you can't see. As long as it's safe to do so, consider using night-lights to light the way to and in your bathroom.

**Keep comfortable.** A bedroom that's too hot or too cold may interfere with sleep. Most people sleep best in a slightly cool room (around 65° F). Replace your mattress and pillows if they're worn or uncomfortable. If aching joints are keeping you awake, ask your doctor about pain relievers. Some people say they are more comfortable sleeping on "memory foam" mattresses and pillows (for example, Tempur-Pedic). See "Musculoskeletal disorders" on page 17 for advice on sleeping positions if you have specific joint pain.

## Try relaxation rituals

Worrying about a problem or a long to-do list can be a recipe for insomnia. Well before you turn in, try writing down your worries and make a list of tasks you want to remember. This "worry journal" may help move these distracting thoughts from your mind.

Closer to bedtime, try comforting rituals that may help lull you to sleep:

- Listen to soft, calming music.
- Take a warm bath.
- Do some easy stretches.
- Read a book or magazine by soft light.

Once you crawl between the sheets, relaxation techniques can help you calm your body and mind. Mindfulness meditation has also proven helpful for battling insomnia. This type of meditation involves focusing on your breathing and then bringing your mind's attention to the present without drifting into concerns about the past or future. To learn more about mindfulness meditation, try one of the free guided recordings by Dr. Ronald Siegel, an assistant professor of psychology at Harvard Medical School and faculty editor

## Screening out blue light: Does it help?

Many people have replaced their incandescent light bulbs with light-emitting diode (LED) and compact fluorescent bulbs, which have the benefit of being more energy-efficient, but the downside of producing more blue light. Electronic devices such as televisions, laptops, and cellphones also emit blue light.

Nighttime exposure to blue light, the shortest of the visible wavelengths, suppresses the brain's production of sleep-inducing melatonin. That means using a blue light–emitting device close to bedtime—whether you're reading a book on a tablet or bingeing your favorite TV series on a laptop—can make it harder for you to fall asleep. Blue light exposure tends to suppress REM sleep as well.

*Exposure to blue light at night can make it harder to fall asleep.*

Short of dimming all the lights and turning off electronic devices, what can you do? One option is to buy a pair of blue light–blocking glasses, which have been shown to improve sleep in a number of studies. According to a 2016 review in *Consumer Reports* magazine that tested three brands of these specialty glasses, only one, Uvex Skyper safety eyewear (orange tinted), cut out almost all blue light. But as the article notes, these glasses do not claim to be medical devices and as such, they are not regulated by the FDA.

Another option is to install an app on your device that automatically shifts the screen color toward warmer hues (that is, reds and yellows) after sundown. However, a small study found that using one of these apps (called NightShift, available on iPhone) did not appear to help, as melatonin levels were still suppressed when people used the app.

© InnerVisionPRO | Getty Images

of the Harvard Special Health Report *Positive Psychology*. The recordings are available at www.mindfulness-solution.com. Many other apps, such as Headspace and Buddhify, are available for downloading on your smartphone, so you can practice any place you like. Try a few to see if one resonates for you.

## Table 3: Caffeine content in common drinks

| DRINK | SERVING SIZE | CAFFEINE (MILLIGRAMS) |
|---|---|---|
| Starbucks coffee | 12 ounces | 235 |
| 5-Hour Energy | 1.9 ounces | 208 |
| Red Bull | 12 ounces | 111 |
| Lipton Pure Leaf Iced Tea | 18.5 ounces | 60 |
| Coca-Cola, Coke Zero, or Diet Pepsi | 12 ounces | 35 |
| Decaf coffee from Dunkin' Donuts, Panera, or Starbucks | 16 ounces | 15–25 |
| Lipton decaffeinated tea, brewed, black or green | 8 ounces | 5 |
| 7-Up or Sprite | 12 ounces | 0 |

*Source: Center for Science in the Public Interest.*

time you went to bed and woke up every day—preferably for two weeks to a month. Include entries for any medications you took, time and quantity of caffeine or alcohol consumption, when and how long you exercised, what time you stopped looking at any electronic devices or TV shows, and any stresses you encountered during the day. All of these can affect sleep. Also note how well you slept each night, whether you awakened during the night, and, if so, for how long.

## Stick to a schedule

A regular sleep schedule keeps the circadian sleep/wake cycle synchronized. People with the most regular sleep habits report the fewest problems with insomnia and the least depression. Experts advise getting up at about the same time every day, even after a late-night party or fitful sleep.

Limit the time you spend in bed. If you don't fall asleep within 20 to 30 minutes or if you wake up and can't fall back to sleep within that amount of time, get out of bed and do something relaxing until you feel sleepy again. Regardless of how well (or poorly) you slept, get out of bed at your regular time each morning to keep your circadian cycle synchronized.

## Negotiate naps, if needed

If your goal is to sleep longer at night, napping is a bad idea. Your total daily sleep need stays constant, so naps take away from evening sleep. But if your goal is to be more

alert during the day, a nap built into your daily schedule may be just the thing. If you have insomnia and feel anxious about getting enough sleep, then a short, scheduled nap may help you sleep better at night by alleviating that anxiety.

If possible, nap soon after lunch. People who snooze later in the afternoon tend to fall into a deeper sleep, which causes greater disruption at night. An ideal nap lasts no longer than 30 to 40 minutes, and even a 15- to 20-minute nap has significant alertness benefits. Shorten or eliminate naps that produce lingering grogginess.

## Keep a sleep diary

A sleep diary may help you uncover clues about what's disturbing your sleep. For example, you may realize that certain habits (like what you eat or drink or when you exercise) are affecting your slumber.

To keep a sleep diary, note what

## Curb caffeine

Caffeine, which is found in coffee, tea, sodas, and other beverages (see Table 3, above), keeps you awake by blocking adenosine, a brain chemical that helps you fall asleep. For some people, a single cup of coffee in the morning means a sleepless night. Caffeine can also interrupt sleep by increasing your need to get up to urinate at night.

If you have insomnia, avoid caffeine as much as possible, since its effects can last for many hours. Because caffeine withdrawal can cause headaches, irritability, and extreme fatigue, some people find it easier to cut back gradually than to go cold turkey. Those who can't or don't want to give up caffeine should avoid it after 2 p.m., or noon if they are especially caffeine-sensitive.

## Nix nightcaps

Alcohol depresses the nervous system, so an alcoholic drink makes some people fall asleep more quickly. But the sleep won't necessarily be very good. Alcohol suppresses REM sleep, and the soporific effects disappear after a few hours. Drinkers have frequent awakenings and sometimes frightening dreams. Alcohol is responsible for up to 10% of chronic insomnia cases. Also, because alcohol relaxes throat muscles and interferes with brain control mechanisms, it can worsen snoring and other nocturnal breathing problems, sometimes to a dangerous extent.

Drinking during one of the body's intrinsic sleepy times—midafternoon or at night—will make a person more drowsy than imbibing at other times of day. Even one drink can make a sleep-deprived person drowsy. If you're driving a car, the combination significantly increases your chances of having an accident.

## Quit tobacco

Nicotine is a potent stimulant that speeds your heart rate, raises your blood pressure, and stimulates fast brain-wave activity that keeps you awake. If you're addicted to nicotine, a few hours without it is enough to induce withdrawal symptoms; the craving can even wake a smoker at night. People who kick the habit fall asleep more quickly and wake less often during the night. Sleep disturbance and daytime fatigue may occur during the initial withdrawal from nicotine. But even during this period, many former users report improvements in sleep. If you continue to use tobacco, avoid smoking or chewing it for at least one to two hours before bedtime.

## Energize with exercise (but not at night)

Walking, jogging, swimming, or any type of exercise that gets your heart pumping faster provides three important sleep benefits: you fall asleep faster, you spend more time in deep sleep, and you awaken less often during the night. Exercise seems to be of particular benefit to older people. In one study, physically fit older men fell asleep in less than half the time it took for sedentary men, and they woke up less often during the night.

Studies also suggest that even gentle exercise, such as stretching and toning, can help people sleep better. Consider trying yoga or tai chi, a stylized martial arts practice that features a series of slow, flowing motions and deep, slow breathing.

Exercise is the only proven way for healthy adults to boost the amount of deep sleep they get. Research shows that older men and women who report sleeping normally can still increase the amount of time they spend in deep sleep if they do some form of aerobic activity.

Exercising outdoors in the morning is ideal, because bright, natural daylight can help set your natural circadian rhythms. Try to avoid exercise within two hours of bedtime because exercise is stimulating and can make it harder to fall asleep.

## Watch when and what you eat and drink

A grumbling stomach can be distracting enough to keep you awake, so if you're hungry right before bed, eat a small healthy snack, such as an apple with a slice of cheese or a few whole-wheat crackers, to satisfy you until breakfast.

But an overly full belly may be even more disrupting. Avoid eating a big meal within two to three hours of bedtime. And steer clear of foods that contribute to acid reflux (heartburn), as lying down can provoke or worsen the problem. Common culprits include coffee, chocolate, alcohol, peppermint, and fatty foods. If you're prone to acid reflux, elevate your upper body with an under-mattress wedge or blocks placed under the bed's legs. Over-the-counter and prescription drugs that suppress stomach acid secretion can also help. Finally, if you sleep on your right side, try to sleep on your left side instead, as several studies suggest that sleeping on your right side aggravates heartburn.

Even if you're careful to avoid caffeinated or alcoholic beverages, drinking too much of any fluid too close to bedtime may cause you to wake up to use the bathroom. ◗

# Medical conditions that disrupt sleep

People who feel they sleep perfectly well may still be troubled by excessive daytime sleepiness because of a variety of underlying medical illnesses. Common conditions often associated with sleep disturbances include breathing problems, diabetes, heart disease, musculoskeletal disorders, kidney disease, mental illness, neurological disorders, and thyroid disease. The stress of chronic illness can also cause insomnia and daytime drowsiness. In addition, a number of prescription and over-the-counter medications used to treat these and other health problems can impair sleep quality and quantity (see Table 4, page 18).

## Breathing problems

Obstructive sleep apnea and central sleep apnea are two serious health conditions in which breathing stops or becomes shallower many times each night, causing the sleeper to rouse, if not completely awaken. These are discussed in greater detail later in the report (see pages 32 and 36, respectively).

However, apnea is not the only breathing issue that can rob a person of sleep. Asthma can also present problems. Circadian-related changes in the tone of the muscles surrounding the airways can cause the airways to constrict during the night, raising the potential for nocturnal asthma attacks that rouse the sleeper abruptly. Breathing difficulties or fear of having an attack may make it more difficult to fall asleep, as can the use of steroids, theophylline (Theo-24, Uniphyl), or other breathing medications that also have a stimulating effect, similar to that of caffeine. People with untreated and undertreated asthma may experience frequent awakenings when they cough, wheeze, or feel short of breath.

People who have emphysema or chronic bronchitis—two diseases that are grouped together under the rubric of chronic obstructive pulmonary disorder (COPD)—may also have difficulty falling and staying asleep because of excess sputum production, shortness of breath, and coughing.

## Diabetes

Night sweats, a frequent need to urinate, or symptoms of hypoglycemia (low blood sugar) often rouse people with diabetes whose blood sugar levels are not well controlled. Tight glucose control will reduce these symptoms. If diabetes has damaged nerves in the legs, nighttime movements or pain may also disturb sleep and require medication for relief and to improve sleep.

## Heart disease

People with heart failure may awaken during the night feeling short of breath because extra body fluid accumulates around their lungs when they're lying down. Placing blocks under the head of the bed to elevate the upper body may help. Sufferers can also be awakened just as they are falling asleep by an abnormal breathing pattern called Cheyne-Stokes respiration, a type of central sleep apnea that is characterized by a series of increasingly deep breaths followed by a brief cessation of breathing. Sleep medications known as benzodiazepines (see page 24) help some people stay asleep, but others may need to use supplemental oxygen or a positive airway pressure (PAP) device that increases pressure in the upper airway and chest cavity.

Coronary artery disease can cause sleep problems, too. The natural fluctuations in hormone secretion reflecting circadian rhythms may trigger angina (chest pain), arrhythmia (irregular heartbeat), or even a heart attack while asleep. Obstructive sleep apnea, which also disturbs sleep, increases the risk of developing coronary artery disease and arrhythmias, setting up a vicious cycle.

## Musculoskeletal disorders

Arthritis pain can make it hard for people to fall asleep and to resettle when they shift positions. In addi-

## Table 4: Medications that may affect sleep

A number of drugs steal sleep, while others may cause unwanted drowsiness. This table includes the most common offenders. Your doctor may be able to suggest alternatives that do not disrupt sleep.

| MEDICATION TYPE | USED TO TREAT | COMMON EXAMPLES | POSSIBLE EFFECT ON SLEEP AND DAYTIME FUNCTIONING |
|---|---|---|---|
| Beta blockers* | High blood pressure, heart rhythm problems, angina | metoprolol (Lopressor), pindolol (Visken), propranolol (Inderal) | Insomnia, nighttime awakenings, nightmares |
| Clonidine | High blood pressure; sometimes prescribed off-label for alcohol withdrawal, smoking cessation, or other health problems | clonidine (Catapres) | Daytime drowsiness and fatigue, disrupted REM sleep; less commonly, restlessness, early morning awakening, nightmares |
| Corticosteroids | Inflammation, asthma | prednisone | Daytime jitters, insomnia, decreased REM sleep |
| Diuretics | High blood pressure | chlorothiazide (Diuril), chlorthalidone (Hygroton), hydrochlorothiazide (Esidrix, HydroDiuril, others) | Increased nighttime urination, painful calf cramps during sleep |
| Medications containing alcohol | Cough, cold, and flu | Contac Cold and Flu, Nyquil Cough, many others | Suppressed REM sleep, disrupted nighttime sleep |
| Medications containing caffeine | Decreased alertness | Caffedrine, NoDoz, Vivarin | Wakefulness that may last up to seven hours |
| | Headaches and other pain | Anacin, Excedrin, Midol | |
| Nicotine replacement products | Smoking | nicotine patches (Nicoderm), gum (Nicorette), nasal spray or inhalers (Nicotrol), and lozenges (Commit) | Insomnia, disturbing dreams |
| Sedating antihistamines** | Cold and allergy symptoms | chlorpheniramine (Chlor-Trimeton), diphenhydramine (Benadryl) | Drowsiness |
| | Motion sickness | dimenhydrinate (Dramamine) | |
| Selective serotonin reuptake inhibitors (SSRIs) | Depression, anxiety | fluoxetine (Prozac), paroxetine (Paxil), sertraline (Zoloft) | Decreased REM sleep, daytime fatigue |
| Sympathomimetic stimulants | Attention deficit disorder | dextroamphetamine and amphetamine (Adderall), methylphenidate (Ritalin, Concerta) | Difficulty falling asleep, decreased REM and non-REM deep sleep |
| Theophylline | Asthma, chronic obstructive pulmonary disease (COPD) | theophylline (Slo-bid, Theo-Dur, others) | Wakefulness similar to that caused by caffeine |
| Thyroid hormone | Hypothyroidism | levothyroxine (Levoxyl, Synthroid, others) | Difficulty falling asleep, fragmented sleep, insomnia (at higher doses) |

*Some beta blockers do not affect sleep; they include atenolol (Tenormin) and sotalol (Betapace).
**These medications are also found in over-the-counter sleep aids.

tion, treatment with corticosteroids frequently causes insomnia. You may find it helpful to take aspirin or a nonsteroidal anti-inflammatory drug (NSAID) just before bedtime, but because of potential side effects, check with your doctor before taking it regularly. Try these sleeping positions to help ease problems with specific joints:

- **Neck:** Sleep with a single flat pillow to place the neck in the most neutral position, avoiding extremes of rotation and sideways bending. Avoid sleeping on your stomach; instead, sleep on your back or side.

- **Low back:** Sleep on your back or side with your knees and hips both flexed to about 90 degrees. This position can relieve pressure on lumbar discs for people with degenerative disc disease or disc herniation. Using a heating pad at bedtime can also help relieve pain.

- **Knee:** Sleep with a pillow between your legs to reduce strain on the joint.

- **Hip:** Sleep on your side with a pillow between your legs, or sleep on your back to avoid a position that rotates the hip.

People with fibromyalgia—a condition characterized by painful ligaments and tendons—are likely to wake in the morning still feeling fatigued and as stiff and achy as a person with arthritis. Researchers who analyzed the sleep of fibromyalgia sufferers have found that at least half have abnormal deep sleep, in which slow (delta) brain waves are mixed with faster (alpha) waves that are usually associated with relaxed wakefulness, a pattern called alpha-delta sleep. In one study, 62 people with fibromyalgia received treatment for six weeks with either the NSAID naproxen (Aleve, Naprosyn), the tricyclic antidepressant amitriptyline (Elavil, Endep), both drugs, or a placebo. Almost half of those who took low doses of amitriptyline reported sleeping and feeling better.

## Kidney disease

Kidney disease can cause waste products to build up in the blood and can result in insomnia or symptoms of restless legs syndrome. Although researchers aren't sure why, kidney dialysis or transplant does not always return sleep to normal.

## Mental illness

Almost all people with anxiety or depression have trouble falling asleep and staying asleep. In turn, not being able to sleep may become a focus of ongoing fear and tension, causing further sleep loss.

**General anxiety.** Severe anxiety, formally known as generalized anxiety disorder, is a mental illness characterized by persistent, nagging feelings of worry, apprehension, or uneasiness. These feelings are either unusually intense or out of proportion to the real troubles and dangers of a person's everyday life. People with the disorder typically experience excessive, persistent worry every day or almost every day for a period of six months or more. Common symptoms include trouble falling asleep, trouble staying asleep, and not feeling rested after sleep.

**Phobias and panic attacks.** Phobias, which are intense fears related to a specific object or situation, rarely cause sleep problems unless the phobia is itself sleep-related (such as fear of nightmares or of the bedroom). Panic attacks, on the other hand, often strike at night. In fact, the timing of nocturnal attacks helped convince psychiatrists that these episodes are biologically based. Sleep-related panic attacks do not occur during dreaming, but rather in stage N2 and deep sleep, which are free of psychological triggers. In many phobias and panic disorders, recognizing and treating the underlying problem—often with an anti-anxiety medication—may solve the sleep disturbance.

**Depression.** Because almost 90% of people with serious depression experience insomnia, a physician evaluating a person with insomnia will consider depression as a possible cause. Waking up too early in the morning is a hallmark of depression, and some depressed people have difficulty falling asleep or sleep fitfully throughout the whole night. In chronic, low-grade depression, insomnia or sleepiness may be the most prominent symptom. Laboratory studies have shown that people who are depressed spend less time in deep sleep and may enter REM sleep more quickly at the beginning of the night.

**Bipolar disorder.** Disturbed sleep is a prominent feature of bipolar disorder (manic-depressive illness). Sleep loss may worsen or induce manic symptoms or temporarily alleviate depression. During a manic episode, a person may not sleep at all for several days. After that, a "crash" may occur, during which the person spends most of the next few days in bed.

**Schizophrenia.** Some people with schizophrenia sleep very little when they enter an acute phase of their illness. Between episodes, their sleep patterns are likely to improve, although many schizophrenics rarely obtain a normal amount of deep sleep.

## Neurological disorders

Brain and nerve disorders can cause sleep problems.

**Dementia.** Alzheimer's disease and other forms of dementia may disrupt sleep regulation and other brain functions. Wandering, disorientation, and agitation during the evening and night, a phenomenon known as "sundowning," can require constant supervision and place great stress on caregivers. In such cases, small doses of antipsychotic medications such as haloperidol (Haldol) and thioridazine (Mellaril) are more helpful than benzodiazepine drugs.

**Epilepsy.** People with epilepsy are twice as likely as others to suffer from insomnia. Brain-wave distur-

## Coping with frequent nighttime urination

Nocturia—the need to get up frequently to urinate during the night—is a common cause of sleep loss, especially among older adults. It affects nearly two-thirds of adults ages 55 to 84 at least a few nights per week. A mild case causes a person to wake up at least twice during the night; in severe cases, a person may get up as many as five or six times.

Nocturia becomes more common with age. As you grow older, your ability to concentrate urine (i.e., to remove water from the fluid going into the kidneys) decreases, causing you to produce a higher volume of urine. Also, the bladder tends to lose holding capacity, leading to more frequent emptying.

Older people are also more likely to suffer from medical problems affecting the bladder. Nocturia has numerous possible other causes, including some of the disorders mentioned in this report (heart failure, diabetes), other medical conditions (urinary tract infection, an enlarged prostate, liver failure, multiple sclerosis, sleep apnea), and medication (especially diuretics). Some cases are caused or worsened by excessive fluid intake after dinner, especially drinks containing alcohol or caffeine.

Therapies fall into three categories: behavioral interventions, medication, and treatments to correct medical causes. The first step is to try to identify the cause and correct it. If that doesn't work, behavioral approaches such as cutting down on how much you drink in the two hours before bedtime, especially caffeine and alcohol, may do the trick. If you take diuretics to lower your blood pressure in the evening, ask your doctor about switching to a morning-only dose, as these drugs cause frequent urination. If the nocturia persists, your doctor may prescribe a drug to treat an overactive bladder. The most commonly used is desmopressin (DDAVP, Stimate), which mimics some of the action of the antidiuretic hormone. If the problem stems from increased contractions of the bladder, relaxant agents such as tolterodine (Detrol) and oxybutynin (Ditropan, Oxytrol) can help.

---

bances that cause seizures can also cause deficits in deep sleep or REM sleep. Antiseizure drugs can produce similar changes at first, but tend to correct these sleep disturbances when used for a long time. About one in four people with epilepsy has seizures that occur mainly at night, leading to disturbed sleep and daytime sleepiness. Sleep deprivation can also trigger a seizure, a phenomenon that's been noted in college infirmaries during exam periods, as some students suffer their first seizures after staying up late to study.

**Headaches, strokes, and tumors.** People who are prone to headaches should try to avoid sleep deprivation, as lack of sleep can promote headaches. Both cluster headaches and migraines may be related to changes in the size of blood vessels leading to the cortex of the brain; pain occurs when the walls of the blood vessels dilate. Researchers theorize that as the body catches up on missed sleep, it spends more time in delta sleep, when vessels are most constricted, making the transition to REM sleep more dramatic and likely to induce a headache. Headaches that awaken people are often migraines, but some migraines can be relieved by sleep.

Sleepiness coupled with dizziness, weakness, headache, or vision problems may signal a serious problem such as a brain tumor or stroke, which requires immediate medical attention.

**Parkinson's disease.** Almost all people with Parkinson's disease have insomnia. Just getting in and out of bed can be a struggle, and the disease often disrupts sleep. Some arousals are from the tremors and movements caused by the disorder, and others seem to result from the disorder itself. Treatment with sleeping pills may be difficult because some drugs can worsen Parkinson's symptoms. Some people who take drugs containing levodopa (such as Sinemet), the mainstay of Parkinson's treatment, develop severe nightmares; others experience disruption of REM sleep. However, the use of these medications at night is important to maintain the mobility needed to change positions in bed. A bed rail or an overhead bar (known as a trapeze) may make it easier for people with Parkinson's to move about and, therefore, lead to better sleep.

### Thyroid disease

An overactive thyroid (hyperthyroidism) overstimulates the nervous system, making it hard to fall asleep, and may cause night sweats, leading to nighttime arousals. Feeling cold and sleepy is a hallmark of an underactive thyroid (hypothyroidism). Because thyroid function affects every organ and system in the body, the symptoms can be wide-ranging and sometimes difficult to decipher. Checking thyroid function requires only a simple blood test, so if you notice a variety of unexplained symptoms, ask your doctor for a thyroid test. ▼

# Insomnia

If you suffer from insomnia, you may be plagued by trouble falling asleep, unwelcome awakenings during the night, and fitful sleep. You may feel drowsy during the day, yet still be unable to nap. You may frequently be anxious, irritable, forgetful, and unable to concentrate.

Although it's the most common sleep disturbance, insomnia is not a single disorder, but rather a general symptom like fever or pain. Finding a remedy requires uncovering the cause. Nearly half of insomnia cases stem from psychological or emotional problems. Stressful events, mild depression, or an anxiety disorder can keep you awake at night. With proper treatment of the underlying cause, the insomnia usually recedes. If it doesn't, additional treatment focusing on sleep may help. The two main approaches to treating insomnia—behavioral therapy and medications—are both effective. But behavioral therapy has been shown to last longer and doesn't have the side effects that can occur with medications.

## Types of insomnia

One way doctors classify insomnia is by its duration. Insomnia is considered transient if it lasts only a few days, short-term if it continues for a few weeks, and chronic if the problem persists.

The causes of transient or short-term insomnia are usually apparent to the sufferer—the death of or separation from a loved one, nervousness about an upcoming event (such as a wedding, public speaking engagement, or move), jet lag, or discomfort from an illness or injury. Chronic insomnia may be caused by a number of medications or medical conditions (see "Medical conditions that disrupt sleep," page 17). In these instances, treating the condition or changing the medication may relieve the insomnia.

One common form of persistent sleeplessness is conditioned (learned) insomnia. After a few sleepless

Don't spend hours in bed not sleeping. If you haven't fallen asleep in 20 to 30 minutes, move to another room and do something relaxing until you feel sleepy. Then return to bed.

nights, some people learn to associate the bedroom with being awake. Taking steps to compensate for sleep deprivation—napping, drinking coffee, having a nightcap, or forgoing exercise—only fuels the problem. As insomnia worsens, anxiety regarding the insomnia may also worsen, leading to a vicious cycle in which fears about sleeplessness and its consequences become the primary cause of the insomnia.

Trouble falling asleep is known as sleep-onset insomnia. Yet another type of insomnia is known as sleep-maintenance insomnia. It refers to difficulty staying asleep, and in particular, waking too early and struggling to get back to sleep. People with certain health problems, including pain, depression, and obstructive sleep apnea, may be more prone to this type of insomnia.

## First-line treatment: Behavioral changes

For chronic insomnia, the first step is changing your lifestyle and habits. The sleep hygiene techniques described earlier in this report are a good begin-

© monkeybusinessimages | Getty Images

ning (see "Practical tips for sounder sleep," page 13). In addition, your doctor will want to pinpoint habits that keep you up at night. A sleep specialist trained in behavioral medicine can help people with learned insomnia replace their bad habits with positive ones. Some people may start sleeping better with behavior changes alone. But others may also need to change their thoughts and beliefs about their sleeping habits—a process referred to as cognitive restructuring.

The combination of all of these techniques is known as cognitive behavioral therapy for insomnia (CBT-i). Following are some of the techniques that are included under this broad umbrella.

### Sleep restriction

People with insomnia often spend more time in bed, hoping this will lead to sleep. In reality, spending less time in bed—a technique known as sleep restriction—promotes more restful sleep and helps make the bedroom a welcome sight instead of a torture chamber. As you learn to fall asleep quickly and sleep soundly, the time in bed is slowly extended until you obtain a full night's sleep.

Some sleep experts suggest starting with six hours at first, or whatever amount of time you typically sleep at night. Setting a rigid early morning waking time often works best. If the alarm is set for 7 a.m., a six-hour restriction means that no matter how sleepy you are, you must stay awake until 1 a.m. Once you are sleeping well during the allotted six hours, you can add another 15 or 30 minutes, then repeat the process until you're getting a healthy amount of sleep.

### Stimulus control

Developed in the 1970s, this technique (also known as reconditioning) trains people with insomnia to associate the bedroom with sleep instead of sleeplessness and frustration. These are the rules:

- Use the bed only for sleeping or sex.
- Don't spend time in bed not sleeping. Go to bed only when you're sleepy. If you're unable to sleep, move to another room and do something relaxing. Stay up until you are sleepy, then return to bed. If sleep does not follow quickly, repeat.
- During the reconditioning process, get up at the same time every day and do not nap, regardless of how much sleep you got the night before.

Another related tip: Cover up your clock or face it away from your view, because watching or checking a clock while you're trying to fall asleep can be frustrating.

### Relaxation techniques

For some people with insomnia, a racing or worried mind is the enemy of sleep. In others, physical tension is to blame. Techniques to quiet a racing mind or a tense body—such as meditation, breathing exercises, progressive muscle relaxation, and biofeedback—can be learned in behavioral therapy sessions or from books or classes.

Progressive muscle relaxation, which involves progressively tensing and relaxing your muscles starting with your feet and working your way up your body, is a tried-and-true, drug-free technique for achieving both physical and mental relaxation. A typical approach is this:

**1** Lie on your back in a comfortable position. Put a pillow under your head if you like, or place one under your knees to relax your back. Rest your arms, with palms up, slightly apart from your body. Feel your shoulders relax.

**2** Take several slow, deep breaths through your nose. Exhale with a long sigh to release tension.

**3** Focus on your feet and ankles. Are they painful or tense? Tighten the muscles briefly to feel the sensation. Let your feet sink into the floor or the bed. Feel them getting heavy and becoming totally relaxed. Let them drop from your consciousness.

**4** Slowly move your attention through different parts of your body: your calves, thighs, lower back, hips, and pelvic area; your middle back, abdomen, upper back, shoulders, arms, and hands; your neck, jaw, tongue, forehead, and scalp. Feel your body relax and your lungs gently expand and contract. Relax any spots that are still tense. Breathe softly.

**5** If thoughts distract you, gently ignore them and return your attention to your breathing. Your worries and thoughts will be there when you are ready to acknowledge them.

© GoodLifeStudio | Getty Images

Ironically, reducing the time you spend in bed—a practice known as sleep restriction—can help you overcome insomnia. Setting a rigid early morning waking time can help you feel sleepy at bedtime.

Another way to release physical tension and relax more effectively is to use biofeedback. This approach involves using equipment that monitors involuntary body states (such as muscle tension or hand temperature) and makes you aware of them. Immediate feedback helps you see how various thoughts or relaxation maneuvers affect tension, enabling you to learn how to gain voluntary control over the process. Biofeedback is usually done under professional supervision.

## Cognitive restructuring

Cognitive restructuring teaches people new ways of thinking about and then doing things. Cognitive restructuring has proved helpful in treating addictions, phobias, and anxiety—as well as insomnia.

Cognitive restructuring for insomnia aims to change negative thoughts and beliefs about sleep into positive ones. People with insomnia tend to become preoccupied with sleep and apprehensive about the consequences of poor sleep. This worry makes relaxing and falling asleep nearly impossible—a phenomenon some experts refer to as "insomniaphobia." The basic tenets of this therapy include setting realistic goals and learning to let go of inaccurate thoughts that can interfere with sleep.

Here are some common types and examples of these thoughts:

- **Misattributions:** "When I make a mistake at work, it's because I did not sleep well the night before."
- **Hopelessness:** "I'll never get a decent night's rest."
- **Unrealistic goals:** "I have to get eight hours of sleep without interruption every night" or "I have to fall asleep before my spouse does."
- **Exaggerating consequences:** "If I don't get to sleep soon, I'll embarrass myself at tomorrow's meeting."
- **Performance anxiety:** "It will take me at least an hour to fall asleep."

A therapist helps you replace these maladaptive thoughts with accurate and constructive ones, such as "All my problems do not stem from insomnia," "I stand a good chance of getting a good night's sleep tonight," or "My job does not depend on how much sleep I get tonight." The therapist also provides structure and support while you practice new thoughts and habits. Typically, you meet with the therapist once a week for an hour, for six to eight weeks.

## How well does CBT-i work?

In recent years, CBT-i has been refined and expanded for greater effectiveness.

In a review article in *Annals of Internal Medicine*, researchers combined data from 20 different trials of CBT-i involving more than 1,100 people with chronic insomnia. On average, people treated with CBT-i fell asleep almost 20 minutes faster and spent 30 fewer minutes awake during the night compared with people who didn't undergo CBT-i. These improvements are as good as, or better than, those seen in people who take prescription sleep medications such as zolpidem (Ambien) and eszopiclone (Lunesta). Unlike sleeping pills, CBT-i helps you overcome the underlying cause of your insomnia without unwanted side effects. And unlike medications, CBT-i continues to be effective even after the therapy ends—in one study, up to the entire six months the researchers evaluated. Medications, in contrast, stop working when you stop taking them.

The biggest obstacle to successful treatment with CBT-i is the commitment it requires. Some people fail to complete all the required sessions or to practice the techniques on their own. Internet-based programs might help address that problem. Several small studies suggest that online CBT-i programs that teach people good sleep hygiene, relaxation techniques, and other strategies can help insomniacs sleep better.

One such program, developed at the University of Virginia Center for Behavioral Medicine Research, helped long-term insomniacs boost their sleep efficiency by an average of 16%, and participants were about half as likely to wake up after falling asleep, compared with a control group. Another study documented at least mild improvements in about 80% of people who completed five weeks of online CBT-i, with 35% reporting that their sleep was "much improved" or "very much improved." As of late 2018, the program was only available to current subscribers or people taking part in clinical trials. However, Pear Therapeutics, which has licensed the program, said it was seeking FDA marketing approval.

Another program, Sleepio, is available as an online program or smartphone app. A 2018 study in *JAMA Psychiatry* followed 1,711 people with insomnia for a year. About half were assigned to six 20-minute sessions of the Sleepio program, while others received online information about sleep hygiene. Sleepio improved not only insomnia, but also daytime functioning and overall health. This program is primarily available through employers or health insurers.

More readily accessible is an app called CBT-i Coach, which was developed by the Department of Veterans Affairs and can be downloaded by anyone for free. It has also proved effective in a small study. It can be used on its own but is intended to augment care with a health care professional.

Many health insurance plans cover CBT-i, which falls under mental health coverage. There's only one problem: not many therapists are trained in this specific type of talk therapy. But some insurers are starting to provide access to online CBT-i programs. If you want face-to-face treatment, you can search for certified specialists across the country by going to the websites of the Society for Behavioral Sleep Medicine (go to www.behavioralsleep.org and click "Provider Search") and the American Board of Sleep Medicine (www.absm.org/BSMSpecialists.aspx).

# Prescription medications for insomnia

Prescription medications help some people with insomnia, but it's best to use them at the lowest effective dose and for the shortest possible period of time. These drugs are most appropriate for short-term problems that disrupt sleep, such as traveling across time zones or coping with a death in the family. For longer-term insomnia, behavioral therapies should be tried first, as they are often just as effective and may have longer-lasting benefits—without the side effects of drugs.

Medications to treat insomnia include benzodiazepines, which are also used to treat anxiety; related medications known as nonbenzodiazepines, which selectively target sleep receptors in the brain; and antidepressants, which are typically prescribed in doses lower than those used to treat depression. Two newer sleep drugs target two different brain chemicals—melatonin and orexin—involved in sleep regulation. (For a complete list, see Table 5, page 25.)

## Benzodiazepines

These medications enhance the activity of GABA, a neurotransmitter that calms brain activity. Different benzodiazepines vary in how quickly they take effect and how long they remain active in the body. Taken at night, benzodiazepines can lead to next-day drowsiness and sedation. If your main problem is getting to sleep, your doctor may prescribe one that begins working quickly and is short-acting, such as triazolam (Halcion). If your problem is staying asleep, a drug that lasts longer—such as estazolam (ProSom) or temazepam (Restoril)—may be necessary. These drugs are useful for people with anxiety and insomnia that results from it.

However, benzodiazepines have a number of drawbacks. For one thing, they reduce how much deep sleep (N3 sleep) you get. For another, many people who use benzodiazepines develop tolerance—the need to take more and more of the drug in order to obtain the same effect. After a few weeks, the drugs may no longer promote sleep. Another

*Continued on page 26*

## Table 5: Prescription medications for insomnia

| GENERIC NAME (BRAND NAME) | SIDE EFFECTS | COMMENTS |
|---|---|---|
| **Benzodiazepines (for short-term treatment of insomnia)** | | |
| alprazolam* (Xanax)<br>clonazepam* (Klonopin)<br>diazepam* (Valium)<br>estazolam (ProSom)<br>flurazepam (Dalmane)<br>lorazepam* (Ativan)<br>quazepam (Doral)<br>temazepam (Restoril)<br>triazolam (Halcion) | Clumsiness or unsteadiness, dizziness, lightheadedness, daytime drowsiness, headache | Should be used with caution by people with sleep apnea or other breathing difficulties; not to be used with alcohol or other depressants; tolerance may develop; withdrawal symptoms occur if stopped abruptly.<br><br>Triazolam is a short-acting medication. |
| **Nonbenzodiazepines (for insomnia)** | | |
| eszopiclone (Lunesta)<br>zaleplon (Sonata)<br>zolpidem** (Ambien, Ambien CR) | Headache, daytime drowsiness, dizziness, nausea, drugged feeling | Don't take these medications with alcohol and certain depressants (including antihistamines, muscle relaxants, and sedatives). |
| **Antidepressants (for insomnia, nonrestorative sleep, and depression)** | | |
| **Serotonin modulator**<br>trazodone* (Desyrel) | Dizziness, dry mouth, headache, nausea, constipation or diarrhea, painful erections | Do not take with a monoamine oxidase inhibitor (MAOI) or while recovering from a heart attack. |
| **Selective serotonin reuptake inhibitors (SSRIs)**<br>citalopram* (Celexa)<br>fluoxetine* (Prozac)<br>fluvoxamine* (Luvox)<br>paroxetine* (Paxil)<br>sertraline* (Zoloft) | Dry mouth, drowsiness, dizziness, sexual dysfunction, nausea, diarrhea, headache, jitteriness, sweating, insomnia, weight gain | |
| **Serotonin and norepinephrine reuptake inhibitor (SNRI)**<br>venlafaxine* (Effexor) | Upset stomach, excitement or anxiety, dry mouth, skin sensitivity to sunlight, weight gain, headache | |
| **Tetracyclic**<br>mirtazapine* (Remeron) | Dry mouth, constipation, weight gain, headache, dizziness | |
| **Tricyclics**<br>amitriptyline* (Elavil)<br>doxepin (Sinequan,* Silenor)<br>nortriptyline* (Aventyl, Pamelor)<br>trimipramine* (Surmontil) | Dry mouth, dizziness, constipation, incomplete urination, weight gain, sun sensitivity, sweating, faintness upon standing, increased heart rate, sexual dysfunction | |
| **Melatonin-receptor agonist (for insomnia and circadian rhythm disorders)** | | |
| ramelteon (Rozerem) | Dizziness | May exacerbate depression; not to be used by people who have severe liver damage or who take fluvoxamine (Luvox). |
| **Orexin-receptor antagonist (for insomnia)** | | |
| suvorexant (Belsomra) | Dizziness, headache, unusual dreams, dry mouth, cough | Use for sleep-maintenance insomnia |

*Although the FDA has not approved these drugs for insomnia, physicians have found that they often help people with insomnia and therefore prescribe them. The only antidepressant with FDA approval for insomnia is Silenor. (Sinequan has the same active ingredient, but it does not have approval for this use.)

**See "Nonbenzodiazepines," page 26, for a description of the different formulations of this medication.

*Continued from page 24*

risk is that stopping the medication abruptly after using it for months can cause insomnia that's even worse than the insomnia you had before you started taking the drug (a phenomenon known as rebound). These medications should be discontinued under a doctor's supervision because withdrawal may lead to muscle tension, restlessness, irritability, or, in rare cases, convulsions.

### Nonbenzodiazepines

These medications—which include eszopiclone (Lunesta), zaleplon (Sonata), and zolpidem (Ambien, Edluar, Intermezzo, Zolpimist)—also enhance the sleep-inducing activity of GABA. But while benzodiazepines affect a range of different receptors in the brain, the nonbenzodiazepines act only on the sleep receptors, which means they cause fewer side effects. They also appear to have little or no effect on deep sleep.

While zolpidem and zaleplon are both approved only to treat short-term insomnia (for up to 30 days), eszopiclone is approved to treat insomnia for up to six months. This does not mean eszopiclone is necessarily

superior—just that its manufacturer took the time and expense to conduct studies to show the drug is safe and effective for longer use. The long-term effects of nonbenzodiazepines remain unknown.

All three drugs make you fall asleep quicker, but only eszopiclone and zolpidem lengthen total sleep time. Zaleplon and zolpidem act quickly (within 20 minutes) and, for the most part, wear off before your typical waking time. Zaleplon wears off especially quickly, so it may not keep you asleep the whole night if you take it before bed. But you can take one if you wake up in the middle of the night and can't fall back asleep. Eszopiclone takes a little longer to take effect and also lasts longer. A long-acting version of zolpidem, called Ambien CR, helps with problems with staying asleep as well as falling asleep.

Zolpidem, the most commonly prescribed sleep medication, comes in multiple forms. Most common is a tablet you swallow with water (Ambien). But it also comes as a tablet you place under your tongue (Edluar, Intermezzo) and an oral spray (Zolpimist), which you spray over your tongue. These new formulations are absorbed more quickly, so they may take effect sooner—and are easier to use because you don't need water to take them. Intermezzo contains a lower dose of zolpidem (less than half of the amount in an Ambien tablet), so it wears off in about four hours—a benefit for those who wake up in the middle of the night and need help to fall back asleep. In fact, Intermezzo is the only prescription sleep medication approved for middle-of-the-night awakening.

Zolpidem also has downsides. Some people find it isn't powerful enough to put them to sleep. And it may cause morning grogginess, tolerance, and rebound insomnia, as well as headache, dizziness, nausea, and, in rare cases, sleepwalking and sleep eating (see "Sleeping pills and sleep eating?" at left). In early 2013, the FDA warned that people who take zolpidem can also wake up the next morning with drug levels high enough to impair their ability to drive and do other activities safely—even if they feel wide awake. Experts originally believed zolpidem worked quickly and left the body quickly, too—but new data suggest it takes longer than previously thought for the drug to be eliminated. The highest risk is with

## Sleeping pills and sleep eating?

Several news reports in 2006 drew attention to a strange side effect of zolpidem (Ambien): sleep eating. People were seen foraging for food at night but were unable to remember the episodes in the morning, or they reported finding evidence of a midnight feast with no recollection of the event. Several people even gained quite a lot of weight.

Other unusual side effects seen with Ambien and other forms of zolpidem include sleepwalking, short-term amnesia, and, rarely, sleep driving. Some of the driving cases occurred when people took sleep medication after drinking alcohol. As a result of these incidents, the FDA ordered the drugs' manufacturers to issue strong new label warnings about the risks of unusual behavior and to produce brochures about safe use.

Although rare, these incidents highlight the need for people who use sleep medications to be aware of the potential side effects and to use them properly. Always allow at least eight hours for sleep, use only as directed, and avoid alcohol. If you experience any unusual occurrences, talk to your doctor right away.

the extended-release form (available as a generic or as Ambien CR). Women are particularly vulnerable because they clear zolpidem from their bodies more slowly than men do. All the other forms of zolpidem (except for Intermezzo) may cause the same problem. As a result, the agency has told manufacturers to lower the starting dose of products containing zolpidem, as follows:

- For women, the 10-mg recommended dose for Ambien, Edluar, and Zolpimist should be cut in half to 5 mg; 12.5-mg doses of extended-release zolpidem (Ambien CR) should be cut in half to 6.25 mg.
- For men, clinicians should consider prescribing a 5-mg dose for regular zolpidem and a 6.25-mg dose for the extended-release form.

Yet a 2018 report in *JAMA Internal Medicine* found that unsafe zolpidem use is common. Among the 3.8 million people who had one or more prescriptions for the drug in 2015, 68% were taking the drug for much longer than recommended (sometimes more than six months). And 41% of all zolpidem users took the drug in combination with related drugs, such as benzodiazepines or opioid-based pain relievers. Women were nearly twice as likely to take zolpidem as men, and use increased with age.

In addition, researchers at the Mayo Clinic in Rochester, Minn., found that hospitalized people who take zolpidem have four times the risk of falls compared with those who don't take the sleep aid. The findings, published in the *Journal of Hospital Medicine*, prompted the Mayo Clinic to phase out its use of zolpidem (which is commonly used in hospitals) and rely more on nondrug methods to promote sleep. These include emphasizing quiet, reducing interruptions, and helping people use techniques such as progressive muscle relaxation, guided imagery, and breathing exercises. Guidance on some of these techniques is available via video in hospital rooms.

With any sleep medication, allow for eight hours of sleep, and avoid doing things that demand high levels of alertness first thing in the morning.

## Antidepressants

The only antidepressant with FDA approval to treat insomnia is doxepin (Silenor). Other antidepressants commonly prescribed "off-label" for insomnia include trazodone (Desyrel) and amitriptyline (Elavil, Endep). The medications are typically used at a lower dose than used for treating depression. Studies of depressed people who also have sleep problems show that these medications reduce the time it takes to fall asleep and decrease the number of nighttime arousals. How they work isn't clear, but sleep may result from a sedative effect. In addition, the drugs' ability to ease anxiety and mild depression may make it easier for people with these problems to relax and fall asleep.

The effect of antidepressants on sleep quality varies; in general, they reduce REM sleep but have little impact on deep sleep. Side effects—namely dizziness, dry mouth, upset stomach, weight gain, and sexual dysfunction—are common. These drugs also can increase leg movements during sleep. Some people find certain antidepressants make them feel nervous or restless, so the medication can actually make insomnia worse. It's not clear if these medications lead to tolerance or rebound insomnia. However, some doctors believe antidepressants have fewer side effects and are safer for long-term use than benzodiazepines.

## Melatonin-receptor agonist

Ramelteon (Rozerem) mimics the body's naturally produced melatonin, a hormone that promotes sleep. It stimulates the same receptors as melatonin in the suprachiasmatic nucleus, the part of the brain that controls the circadian cycle of sleep and wakefulness. Ramelteon has a more potent effect than over-the-counter melatonin, which helps some people fall asleep faster and can be used to adjust the circadian sleep phase. Ramelteon takes effect quickly, but it also wears off within hours. For that reason, the drug is approved to treat insomnia for people who have trouble falling asleep at bedtime rather than those who have trouble staying asleep.

Ramelteon's most common side effect is dizziness, and it may also worsen symptoms of depression. People who have severe liver damage or who use the antidepressant fluvoxamine (Luvox) shouldn't take it. Citing clinical studies that found ramelteon did not cause tolerance, dependence, or rebound insomnia,

### ▶ Gadgets that promise better sleep: Worth a try?

In recent years, a number of smartphone apps, gadgets, and specialized devices that pledge to deliver a more satisfying slumber have hit the market, aimed directly to sleep-deprived consumers. They include a range of products, from wristband or mattress sensors that record your movement in bed to specialized lights that claim to help you fall asleep or wake up.

Be aware that there's little research demonstrating the effectiveness of any of these products, which don't require a great deal of evidence to gain marketing approval. There are no known downsides to trying any of them, save for the cost (if any). If you try one but still have troubling symptoms, consult your health care provider.

---

the drug's manufacturer promotes it for long-term use.

The drug may be more likely to benefit older rather than younger people, since people produce less melatonin as they age. However, older people's primary sleep problem tends to be waking up during the night, not falling asleep at the beginning of the night, suggesting ramelteon's usefulness may be limited.

### Orexin-receptor antagonist

Suvorexant (Belsomra) works by blocking orexin (also known as hypocretin)—a neurotransmitter that promotes wakefulness. People with narcolepsy, who experience sudden "sleep attacks," lack orexin-producing cells in their brains—a discovery that led to the development of suvorexant.

Suvorexant should be taken within 30 minutes of going to bed and only if you can devote at least seven hours to sleep. Like some of the nonbenzodiazepines, it can cause next-day drowsiness, in addition to other side effects such as dizziness, headache, and unusual dreams. It may be helpful for treating sleep-maintenance insomnia (when you wake up too early and can't get back to sleep) and for people who are hospitalized.

## Over-the-counter sleep aids

Drugstores carry a bewildering variety of over-the-counter sleep products. But do these products work? And if you try them, should you choose a sleeping pill, an herbal remedy, or a dietary supplement?

### Nonprescription sleeping pills

There is a riot of competing brands, but otherwise these products are remarkably similar. Each one—whether a tablet, capsule, or gelcap—contains an antihistamine as its primary active ingredient. Most over-the-counter sleep aids—including Nytol, Sominex, and others—contain 25 to 50 milligrams (mg) of the antihistamine diphenhydramine. A few, such as Unisom SleepTabs, contain 25 mg of doxylamine, another antihistamine. (Note that antihistamines are also found in pain relievers like Tylenol PM, Excedrin PM, Aleve PM, and Advil PM, which are typically marketed for "occasional sleeplessness associated with minor aches and pains.")

The antihistamines found in these products have a sedating effect and are generally safe when taken as directed for brief time periods. But they can cause nausea and, more rarely, fast or irregular heartbeat, blurred vision, or heightened sensitivity to sunlight. Complications are generally more common in children and in people over age 60. Diphenhydramine blocks the brain chemical acetylcholine, which is essential for normal brain function, and elderly people who take these drugs face a higher risk of cognitive problems, including delirium. Alcohol heightens the effect of these medications, which can also interact adversely with some drugs. Sleep experts generally advise against using these medications for more than brief periods because they are often ineffective and because of the possibility of these side effects.

### Dietary supplements

As with multivitamins and other supplements, the FDA does not regulate these products, so they aren't tested for safety, effectiveness, quality, or accuracy of labeling. One problem with supplements in general is that they often do not contain the amount of the active ingredient stated on the label and may contain other substances not listed.

© PonyWang | Getty Images

There are other potential problems. Although marketed as "natural," these products may contain biologically active substances that can have side effects or interact with other medications or supplements. For example, scientists have identified more than 100 compounds in valerian root. Researchers don't know precisely which of these account for the herb's effect, nor can they say exactly how these or other compounds in valerian might interact with other medications. If you're thinking about using such products (or already do so), be sure to tell your doctor.

Finally, what we know generally comes from small, short-term studies. Thus, most doctors discourage the use of herbal medicines as sleep aids.

Readily available alternative sleep remedies typically include one or more of the following substances.

**Valerian (Valeriana officinalis).** A few studies suggest that valerian is mildly sedating and can help people fall asleep and improve their sleep quality. But a review in the *Journal of Clinical Sleep Medicine* pointed out that most of the studies were small and flawed, and that even the positive studies showed only a mild effect. The most common reported side effects are headaches, dizziness, itching, and gastrointestinal disturbances. Additionally, there can be a problem with the amount of active ingredient you actually get. A report by ConsumerLab.com—a commercial laboratory that periodically tests the quality of herbal remedies—found that nearly a quarter of valerian-based products appeared to contain no valerian whatsoever, and an equal number had less than half the amount claimed on their labels.

**Chamomile.** Tea made from this flower, a member of the daisy family, is a traditional remedy long used to help people relax and become drowsy. Chamomile is both mild and safe, although rare allergic reactions, including bronchial constriction, can occur. If you're allergic to plants in the daisy family, which includes ragweed, you should probably avoid this herb. There are no scientific studies showing chamomile is effective in treating insomnia.

**Synthetic melatonin.** Melatonin is a hormone, produced in the brain at night, that plays a role in regulating sleep and circadian rhythms. Since the 1990s, a synthetic version has been widely available in the United States as a supplement at health food stores and pharmacies. Despite some initial enthusiasm for synthetic melatonin, most subsequent research has been disappointing, finding either minimal benefits or none at all. One analysis that pooled findings from 17 different studies found than taking melatonin helped people fall asleep just four minutes faster and added only 12 minutes to their total sleep time, on average. A review by the federal Agency for Healthcare Research and Quality (AHRQ) concluded that the supplement "is not effective in treating most sleep disorders."

However, a subset of people do appear to benefit: those whose insomnia results from delayed sleep-wake phase disorder (see page 45), a circadian rhythm disorder in which people don't start to feel sleepy until hours after the conventional bedtime. The AHRQ review found that melatonin enables people with this disorder to fall asleep an average of nearly 40 minutes faster than they would with a placebo.

Melatonin only exerts an effect for one to two hours and does not appear to pose any major health risks when taken for a short time. The most commonly reported side effects are nausea, headache, and dizziness. Its long-term effects are unknown. As with other dietary supplements, the amount of active ingredient may vary widely: One Canadian study of 31 melatonin supplements found that 70% of the products contained 10% or less of what was listed on the label. However, one chewable tablet had nearly 9 mg of melatonin when it was supposed to contain just 1.5 mg.

Surprisingly, smaller doses appear to work better than larger ones. If you take synthetic melatonin, do not take more than 3 mg. Often tablets contain up to 5 mg. Because the quality and purity of most over-the-counter melatonin supplements is unknown, be cautious about what you purchase. One option is a brand of prescription-grade melatonin supplements from a company called Pure Encapsulation. This company supplies melatonin to European markets, where the hormone is available only by prescription; they provide the same product in the United States. ▼

# Breathing disorders in sleep

Although relaxed and steady breathing is natural for most sleepers, some people snore so loudly that they literally wake the neighbors. Loud snoring may be a sign of sleep apnea, a life-threatening condition marked by frequent interruptions in breathing. In most cases, however, people who snore only suffer from simple snoring produced when the muscles of the airways relax during sleep—a condition that doesn't cause medical complications but may disrupt the sleep of others nearby.

## Snoring

When you fall asleep, muscles in your airway relax, causing the airway to narrow. Snoring occurs when it narrows too much, causing turbulent airflow. The surrounding tissue vibrates, producing noise. One population study reported that 24% of women and 40% of men were habitual snorers.

If your nasal passages are swollen by a cold, allergies, or a reaction to smoke, you may snore temporarily. But a number of physical characteristics can also contribute to long-term problems with snoring. These include

- a deviated septum (a misalignment of the bone and cartilage that separates the two sides of the nose)
- an elongated soft palate (the fleshy, flexible area toward the back of the roof of the mouth)
- a large uvula (the fleshy piece of tissue that hangs down from the soft palate; a normal-sized one clears the top of the tongue when the mouth is open)
- enlarged tonsils (the small masses of soft tissue on both sides of the back of the throat)
- enlarged adenoids (small lumps of tissue located above the tonsils)
- a very small jaw
- excess fat in the neck area.

The hormones progesterone and estrogen may play a protective role; before menopause, women

Snoring occurs when muscles of the upper aiway relax. Losing even a little weight can help reduce snoring—and give your partner a better night's sleep.

© Wavebreakmedia | Getty Images

snore less than men, but snoring increases among women later in life. Many women snore late in their pregnancies, a phenomenon attributed to hormone-related swelling of airway tissues.

Although snoring is rarely life-threatening, sleep specialists take even simple snoring seriously. A person who snores heavily deserves a thorough examination of the throat, mouth, palate, tongue, and neck and may need to undergo sleep studies.

### Nonsurgical treatments for snoring

Hundreds of devices are marketed as aids for people who wish to stop snoring or improve their nighttime breathing. Some encourage you to sleep on your side; others are dental appliances that try to keep your airway open by preventing your tongue from falling back or by moving your jaw forward. Check with your physician before investing in such a device. There are simple, inexpensive ways to prevent snoring that may serve you just as well.

**Devices.** A variety of simple appliances can help with snoring. Some people snore only when lying on their backs, so devices that encourage lying on the side are helpful (see "Positional aids," page 35). Other people keep air passages open by raising their heads with an extra pillow or by propping up the head of the bed a few inches. Similarly, a pricey new device called Smart Nora gently adjusts your head position if you start snoring. If swollen nasal tissues are the problem, a humidifier or medication such as decongestants or nasal steroids may reduce swelling. Some small studies find that nasal dilators—small adhesive strips you place across the bridge of your nose to open up your nasal passages—may also help reduce the frequency or intensity of snoring.

**Lifestyle changes.** Doctors usually encourage overweight snorers to lose weight. Dropping even just a little weight (5% to 10% of your body weight) can make a difference. If you smoke, quitting may also help alleviate snoring, since the irritation causes swelling of airway tissues. In addition, it makes sense to forgo alcohol, sleeping pills, and tranquilizers, all of which decrease muscle tone.

**Oral devices.** Oral appliances are another option. These are designed to increase the size of your upper airway, either by pushing the jaw forward, changing the position of the soft palate (the fleshy, back area of the upper mouth), retracting the tongue, or a combination of those mechanisms. Typically bought over the counter, these are different from the custom-made appliances dentists use to treat more significant sleep-related breathing problems.

## Surgical treatments for snoring

If your problem is caused by a deviated septum, large tonsils, or enlarged adenoids, surgery may be required. These procedures are quite straightforward and can be quite helpful. In extreme cases, physicians may recommend more extensive surgery, similar to that used to treat sleep apnea. But because those procedures are so invasive and may not have lasting benefits, they should be used as a last resort.

**Laser surgery.** For this procedure, called laser-assisted uvulopalatoplasty (LAUP), an ear, nose, and throat specialist (ENT) uses a carbon dioxide laser to shorten the uvula and to make small cuts in the soft palate on either side of the uvula. As these nicks heal, the surrounding tissue pulls tighter and stiffens. Because snoring results from the flapping of loose tissue at the back of the soft palate, it is less likely to occur when the tissue is smaller and stiffer. Afterward, people usually have a sore throat for about a week. After five weeks of healing, the treatment may be repeated if snoring persists. Three or four procedures (which are done in a doctor's office) may be needed.

While LAUP can be quite effective in stopping snoring, the technique doesn't appear to ease apnea and may not be covered by insurance. What's more, this procedure can be dangerous for people with undiagnosed apnea because it removes the warning signal of this breathing disorder, so be sure you have a physician rule out sleep apnea before undergoing LAUP.

**Somnoplasty.** Also known as radiofrequency tissue volume reduction, this procedure was first approved to treat snoring but later became an option for obstructive sleep apnea. An ENT delivers radiofrequency waves through the tips of tiny needles inserted into the obstructive tissue to shrink it. Somnoplasty takes only a few minutes to perform and doesn't cause bleeding, but it may have to be repeated to achieve results. People typically experience some swelling immediately following the procedure; over-the-counter painkillers can usually control any pain.

**Palatal implants.** In this procedure, also known as the Pillar procedure, a surgeon implants up to three matchstick-sized stiffening rods made of polyester into the soft palate. The rods help keep the palate from collapsing, limiting obstruction of the back of the throat when a person falls asleep. They may improve symptoms, but only if your snoring results from collapse of the palate. The procedure, done under local anesthesia in an office, is reversible. If it causes pain or does not work, the rods can be removed. Sometimes the rods come out on their own, without significant discomfort.

# Sleep apnea

Sleep apnea is a serious health condition in which breathing stops or becomes shallower hundreds of times each night. In the most common form, obstructive sleep apnea, the tongue or throat tissues block the airway. Central sleep apnea, in which the brain does not send messages to the muscles that control breathing, accounts for less than 5% of cases.

Untreated, sleep apnea can have devastating consequences. The relentless daytime fatigue that often results may destroy careers, break up marriages, and lead to automobile and workplace accidents. It can even be life-threatening, contributing to the development of high blood pressure, heart failure, and strokes. A *New England Journal of Medicine* study found that sleep apnea doubles a person's risk of suffering a stroke over a seven-year period. Sleep apnea wreaks havoc on the cardiovascular system because the heart must work harder every time the person rouses to open his or her airway, increasing heart rate, blood pressure, and stress hormones. The repeated occurrences over time lead to permanent increases in blood pressure and stress on the heart and cardiovascular system.

Sleep apnea used to be considered uncommon, and it often remained undiagnosed. Physicians rarely checked for it except in the stereotypical patient—an overweight, middle-aged man who snored. But the prevalence has soared over the past two decades, at least in part because of the obesity epidemic. Still, while more than half of the estimated 25 million Americans who have sleep apnea are overweight, many are not. The disorder affects an estimated 25% of men and 10% of women, and the incidence rises with age.

## Obstructive sleep apnea

Obstructive sleep apnea (OSA) occurs when the upper airway is blocked by excess tissue, such as a large uvula, the tongue, the tonsils, fatty deposits in the airway walls, congested nasal passages, or a floppy rim at the back of the palate (see Figure 5, page 33). People with OSA tend to have smaller airway openings than those who don't. A narrow airway makes obstruction all the more likely when airway muscles relax at the onset of sleep.

When the airway is blocked, you cannot breathe. A potentially life-threatening lack of oxygen and buildup of carbon dioxide, as well as increasing efforts to breathe, cause you to wake and gasp loudly for air until blood oxygen levels return to normal. At worst, a person with OSA cannot breathe and sleep at the same time.

Some people with OSA repeat this cycle hundreds of times a night without being fully aware of what is happening. They don't realize how little sleep they're actually getting and may routinely feel sleepy. Others wake up after bouts of apnea and have difficulty getting back to sleep. They assume that insomnia—not a breathing problem—makes them sleepy during the day. The condition can become even more perilous if a person with OSA uses substances that further relax airway muscles or suppress arousal or breathing, such as muscle relaxants, alcohol, and some sleeping pills.

The symptoms and signs of OSA include the following:

- **Grogginess, fatigue, and sleepiness.** People with OSA are often extremely tired during the day, frequently nodding off when they want to stay awake.
- **Loud, disruptive snoring.** Frequent snoring that is loud enough to disturb a bed partner is a hallmark of OSA. The snorer may choke, gasp, or appear to hold his or her breath during sleep.
- **Thick neck.** Men with a neck circumference of 17 inches or more and women with a neck circumference of 16 inches or more are at higher risk. As with snoring, obesity is a major risk factor, since fatty

---

## The STOPBANG test for sleep apnea

A "yes" answer to three or more of these questions suggests you may have sleep apnea. Ask your doctor if you should have a sleep study.

**S — Snore:** Have you been told that you snore?

**T — Tired:** Do you often feel tired during the day?

**O — Obstruction:** Do you know if you briefly stop breathing while asleep, or has anyone witnessed you do this?

**P — Pressure:** Do you have high blood pressure or take medication for high blood pressure?

**B — Body mass index (BMI):** Is your BMI 30 or above? (For a calculator, see www.health.harvard.edu/bmi.)

**A — Age:** Are you 50 or older?

**N — Neck:** Is your neck circumference more than 16 inches (women) or 17 inches (men)?

**G — Gender:** Are you male?

---

deposits surrounding the throat expand as people gain weight, narrowing the airway.

- **High blood pressure.** More than half of people with OSA have high blood pressure, caused by OSA.

OSA occurs on a spectrum. In some cases, the airway is only slightly narrowed, but people must work extra hard to inhale, although they have no significant drop in blood oxygen levels. This extra work wakes them up many times each night, and they may complain of insomnia or daytime sleepiness. The same treatments that help individuals with a fully closed airway are also effective for these cases.

In the past, diagnosing sleep apnea required an overnight stay in a sleep lab. Today, about 60% to 70% of sleep studies for suspected OSA are done with home-based tests. The tests use sensors and other devices that measure your breathing and blood oxygen while you sleep.

## Treatments for obstructive sleep apnea

Treatment for OSA often includes lifestyle changes, which may improve but usually don't fully resolve the condition. For people with mild to moderate OSA, therapies such as dental devices and positional aids may be reasonable alternatives. However, the gold standard (and most commonly used) treatment is positive airway pressure (PAP). Less common treatments include a variety of surgical procedures.

**Lifestyle changes.** Weight loss is the best treatment for weight-related OSA. Experts recommend losing at least 10% of body weight, optimally with the goal of reaching a normal BMI. But weight loss alone doesn't always cure the problem. Also, because losing

▶ **Weight-loss surgery for apnea?**

Bariatric surgery helps extremely obese people lose weight by reducing the size of the stomach. Initial reports suggested that the extreme weight loss following the surgery could effectively "cure" sleep apnea. But subsequent research revealed that while surgical weight loss can reduce the severity of sleep apnea and eliminate the condition in some people, others will still have sleep apnea following surgery and likely need continued treatment.

weight is challenging and takes a long time to achieve, most people with severe symptoms need additional treatment. Sleeping on your side instead of your back can work if you have OSA only while sleeping on your back. Everyone with OSA should avoid alcohol, seda-

## Figure 5: Apnea—and how PAP helps

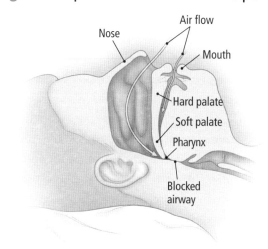

In a person with obstructive sleep apnea, the upper airway—which includes the nose, mouth, and throat—is blocked. In the example above, excess fatty tissue around the soft palate and pharynx is the culprit, but the blockage can occur anywhere along the airway. As a result, air can't enter the lungs, and the resulting drop in oxygen signals the brain to send an emergency "breathe now!" signal that briefly awakens the sleeper and makes him or her gasp for air. These pauses in breathing can last seconds to minutes and can occur up to 100 times per hour.

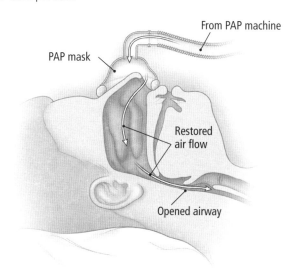

A PAP machine provides a stream of air via a mask that covers the nose. The air pressure prevents the collapse of the airway when the muscles relax during sleep. This allows the person to sleep normally without interruption.

tives, and muscle relaxants. Nasal strips, mechanical dilators, and moisturizing gels and sprays have not been shown to help.

**Positive airway pressure (PAP).** This approach uses one of several models of bedside machines to pump air into a mask that fits snugly over your nose. Blowing air through the nose is the preferred method, unless you have a nasal obstruction or congestion that make it necessary for you to breathe through your mouth. The air pressure opens your airway, preventing collapse when muscles relax during sleep. This allows you to sleep normally and breathe without interruption.

In the original iteration of this device—called continuous positive airway pressure, or CPAP—the air pressure stayed the same as you breathed in and out. But patients often found it uncomfortable to breathe out against a stream of oncoming air. Newer versions may be easier to use. Bi-level PAP (BPAP) delivers air under higher pressure as you inhale and switches to a lower pressure during exhalation. AutoPAP (APAP) takes this improvement a step further by including an internal regulator that moves the pressure up and down according to required pressure needs, using the lowest level of pressure possible.

Many models offer options such as warmed humidified air (which alleviates nasal congestion, skin dryness, and dry mouth) and a timer that slowly builds up pressure after you turn the machine on, to give you time to adapt and fall asleep more easily. There are also a variety of mask styles, allowing you to

The most commonly used treatment for obstructive sleep apnea is an air-pressure device called PAP.

find the one that best fits your face and is most comfortable. Most cover only the nose, but some cover both the nose and the mouth.

People usually try CPAP or BPAP for the first time in a sleep laboratory, so a technician can adjust the air pressure during sleep and let the doctor know what level would be most appropriate for that individual. APAP use doesn't require a sleep laboratory stay, as the machine senses the required pressure and adjusts automatically. Some people adjust to the device without any problem and report that their night in the laboratory is the best night's sleep they've had in years. Others find it difficult at first to tolerate the device and to sleep with the mouth closed. Troubleshooting some common issues with PAP may help (see "Tips for using a PAP machine," page 35).

PAP is covered by most insurance plans. Most people procure the device on a rent-to-buy basis through their insurance companies. You can also order PAP machines online; prices range from $500 to $1,500. PAP generally leads to a great improvement in the amount of time spent in restorative deep sleep, which improves alertness the next day. In many cases, PAP also reduces or eliminates high blood pressure. For some people, PAP is a lifelong treatment.

**Supplemental oxygen.** Given through a tube in the nose (as opposed to a mask placed over the nose), supplemental oxygen can prevent the drops in blood oxygen that accompany airway collapse. However, oxygen does not prevent airway collapse or sleep fragmentation, so it's used in conjunction with other treatments.

**Other devices.** These therapies may be suitable alternatives for people who cannot use PAP machines.

- **Expiratory positive airway pressure.** This technology, marketed under the name Provent, relies on small, circular, single-use valves surrounded by bandage-like adhesive that you place over the opening of each nostril every night. As you breathe in, the valves open. As you breathe out, they partially close. The air that backs up in your airway as you exhale produces the positive pressure that keeps the airway open. Research suggests the device sharply cuts the number of apnea episodes a person has and eliminates OSA in about 50% of

## Tips for using a PAP machine

If you've had trouble using one of these machines, be aware that the newer versions are generally easier to tolerate. These tips may also help:

**Make sure your mask fits properly.** If your mask is too large, tightening the straps that hold it to your face may irritate your skin. If your mask is too small, it won't seal properly, and air may leak out around the edges, possibly into your eyes. Try a different mask if you can't get comfortable with your first choice. Soft strap covers may feel better on your skin. Using a special bed pillow shaped for a PAP mask and tubing may also help.

**Adapt gradually.** At the beginning, use your PAP machine for short stints during the day while you read or watch TV. You'll become more comfortable wearing the mask, so it will feel more natural when you are trying to fall asleep.

**Treat any nose, mouth, or throat discomfort caused by PAP.** Try using a saline or decongestant nasal spray if your nose is dry or stuffy. Many PAP devices have a heated humidifier to ensure that you are breathing warm, moist air through your mask.

**Keep the machine clean.** Because you're breathing air that's processed through the machine, it's important to keep it clean, so that bacteria don't grow inside it. Schedule a regular time to clean your mask, tubing, and headgear once a week, ideally on the same day and time so you don't forget.

---

users. But not everyone finds Provent easy to use, especially people who tend to breathe through the mouth at night, or those who have nasal allergies and a stuffed-up nose. A 30-day supply of the patches costs $65 to $80, and is typically not covered by insurance. It also requires a prescription. But if you can tolerate Provent, the product is far more portable than a PAP device—a special boon for frequent travelers.

- **Dental devices.** These devices reposition the lower jaw and tongue, so that the airway remains open. They are fairly well tolerated and have a success rate of about 50% to 70% for mild to moderate OSA. One type, called a mandibular advancement device, resembles a sports mouth guard and works by pushing the lower jaw forward and down slightly. Another, called a tongue-retaining device, holds the tongue in place to keep the airway as open as possible. These devices are less cumbersome and easier to travel with than PAP. However, they can cause shifting of teeth and problems with the temporomandibular (jaw) joint, so be sure to get the device from a dentist trained in treating people with OSA and get regular follow-ups, including a sleep study done with the device in place to make sure it eliminates the OSA.

- **Positional aids.** Some people only have apnea when they sleep on their backs, so props or devices that encourage them to sleep on their sides sometimes help. Low-tech options include wedge-shaped pillows or a tennis ball sewn into the back of a nightshirt. Another option is a device called Night Shift, which is a small monitor worn on the back of the neck. If you start sleeping on your back, it starts to vibrate with increasing intensity until you change position. It also monitors your sleep quality and how often you snore loudly, and these readings can be uploaded online and shared with your doctor.

**Medications.** Some people with OSA still feel sleepy during the day even after successful treatment. Two medications may help: modafinil (Provigil), which seems to temporarily stop the brain from making neurotransmitters that promote sleep, and a related drug, armodafinil (Nuvigil). Although both can help people with OSA who have trouble staying alert in the day, they do not address the source of the problem and should be used with other treatments, not in place of them.

Intriguingly, researchers in Boston have identified a pair of existing drugs—oxybutynin (Ditropan, Oxytrol; used to treat overactive bladder) and atomoxetine (Strattera; used for attention deficit hyperactivity disorder)—that appear to work together to help maintain the activation of upper airway muscles during sleep. However, the combination is still in testing.

**Surgery.** Most surgical procedures for sleep apnea do not have good success rates. Although some people improve, a sizable percentage don't get better. And some people's symptoms actually worsen—that is, they have more episodes of apnea after the surgery than they had before.

What's behind these poor success rates? Surgeons must deal with a long soft tube of tissue that can collapse at any point—or even at several points—and they can't always predict exactly where it might collapse in the future. Surgery corrects collapse at a single spot, so if a collapse later occurs at a different spot or in several spots, OSA can return.

That's not to say surgery is always a bad idea. If you have OSA, consult with a sleep specialist to review all your options. Then, if you decide on surgery, find a surgeon who has a lot of experience with these procedures to improve your chances for success.

Types of surgery for OSA include the following:

- **Corrective jaw surgery.** Surgery to move the upper or lower jaw forward may enlarge the upper airway for some people with OSA. Centers with specialists in this procedure report success rates up to 90%. However, the procedure requires extensive training and experience. The procedure changes the facial appearance and teeth alignment and requires an extensive recovery period.
- **Uvulopalatopharyngoplasty (UPPP).** This procedure to remove throat tissue helps about 40% to 45% of people with OSA. The rest may need to have further upper airway surgery or use PAP.
- **Upper airway stimulation therapy.** This therapy features a small device that's surgically implanted in the upper chest. The device monitors your breathing and, if needed, stimulates nerves around your tongue and airway to prevent them from collapsing. The FDA-approved system, called Inspire, reduced apnea episodes by 70% in one study.
- **Palatal implants.** Some specialists have started using palatal implants (see page 31) to treat people whose OSA results from an elongated soft palate. It's not yet clear what percentage of people with OSA benefit or how long improvements last.
- **Somnoplasty.** Originally developed to treat snoring, somnoplasty (see page 31) uses radiofrequency waves to shrink obstructive tissues when other treatments have not helped mild OSA. There are limited data supporting its use for OSA.

## Central sleep apnea

Central sleep apnea, or CSA, occurs when breathing centers in the brain fail to send the necessary messages to initiate breathing. Although the airway isn't blocked, the diaphragm and chest muscles stop moving. Shortly, falling blood oxygen and rising carbon dioxide levels set off an internal alarm, triggering you to resume breathing (and often waking you as a result). This rare condition warrants a thorough evaluation to establish the underlying cause, which in turn guides treatment. CSA becomes more common with age and is more frequent and severe in people with heart failure, chronic lung disease, or neurological damage. CSA doesn't cause snoring, but people with this problem are usually aware of waking up during the night and often complain of daytime sleepiness.

Therapy usually involves treating the underlying medical condition that has disrupted breathing. For example, if the CSA is caused by heart failure, medications to treat the heart failure may eliminate the CSA. Some people use PAP and may also receive added oxygen. For people who have CSA only as they begin to fall asleep, a mild sleeping pill may help them fall asleep and stay asleep, solving the breathing problem. Medications such as acetazolamide (Diamox) and theophylline (Theo-24, Uniphyl) benefit some people. ◗

# Movement disorders and parasomnias

Sleep can be disturbed by problems other than insomnia or sleep apnea. Some people are troubled by uncontrollable leg movements, while others experience parasomnias (unusual behaviors such as walking or eating during sleep).

## Movement disorders

Sleepers typically shift position every 15 to 30 minutes, and it's normal for muscles to jerk at the onset of sleep, though the cause of these twitches is a mystery. However, some people have neurological disorders that cause them to move much more than normal. These people may find it impossible to get a restful night's sleep, unless they seek treatment.

### Restless legs syndrome

Restless legs syndrome (RLS) is an exasperating condition that triggers abnormal sensations in the legs (and occasionally the arms) and an irresistible urge to move them. Moving the limbs may bring temporary relief.

RLS affects about 10% of people ages 30 to 70, two-thirds of them women. As many as half of people with RLS note that they have family members with similar symptoms. Each child of an affected person has a 50% chance of inheriting the condition. Researchers have identified specific genes linked to the development of RLS that may account for up to half of all cases of the disorder.

Sleep deprivation is a major problem for people with RLS, as the symptoms are most prominent at night—or, in many cases, occur only at night. RLS symptoms may make it difficult to fall asleep or stay asleep, compelling the person to get in and out of bed many times.

During the day, symptoms are worse when sitting still, and the irresistible urge to move can make it difficult for some people with RLS to take car or plane trips, enjoy a movie, or even hold a desk job. People develop a variety of coping strategies, such as pacing, doing knee bends, rocking, or stretching the leg muscles. Some people get temporary relief by rubbing or squeezing their leg muscles, wrapping their legs in bandages, or applying cold or warm compresses. The daytime symptoms sometimes abate for a few hours, days, or even years.

Because the symptoms sound bizarre or vague—and the need to be constantly mobile seems like nervousness—people with RLS are frequently thought to have psychiatric problems. Children who have RLS are often diagnosed as having attention deficit hyperactivity disorder. Some people report that their symptoms started in adolescence and that adults attributed the problem to growing pains or back trouble.

RLS usually worsens with age (see Figure 6, below). Women may find that symptoms flare up during menstruation, pregnancy, or menopause. At least one in four pregnant women experiences restless legs.

## Figure 6: Prevalence of restless legs syndrome by age

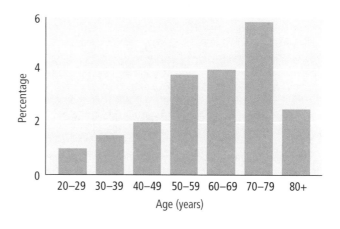

RLS can occur at any age, but it tends to be more common and severe in people over 50.

*Adapted from* Archives of Internal Medicine.

Restless legs can be brought on by alcoholism, iron-deficiency anemia, diabetes, heart failure, or kidney failure. In some people, caffeine, stress, nicotine, fatigue, or prolonged exposure to a cold or very warm environment worsens the symptoms. Certain medications—including antihistamines, antidepressants, or lithium—can also exacerbate RLS.

## Periodic limb movement disorder

A neurological condition called periodic limb movement disorder (PLMD) causes people to kick and jerk their arms and legs throughout the night. Their leg and arm muscles involuntarily contract about every 20 to 40 seconds, so the movement may be repeated hundreds of times a night. These so-called periodic limb movements of sleep can cause brief arousals. PLMD results when they disrupt sleep enough to produce daytime sleepiness.

Most people with RLS also have PLMD, but the reverse is not true. In fact, the two disorders have several key distinctions (see "RLS and PLMD: What's the difference?" below). The health consequences, however, may be similar.

According to some estimates, as many as 30% to 50% of people ages 65 and older have periodic limb movements of sleep. But that figure is based on observations of leg twitches alone, and not all of these people experience the brief, unconscious awakenings that disrupt sleep.

Episodes of limb movements may last only a few minutes, or they may continue for hours, with intervals of sound sleep in between. They usually don't occur continuously throughout the night, but cluster in the first half of the night and occur mainly during non-REM sleep. Instead of proceeding smoothly through all the sleep stages in regular cycles, people with PLMD awaken for a few seconds at a time (generally without realizing it) and frequently skip back to the lighter stages of sleep. Unless a bed partner complains, people with PLMD are often oblivious to the movements and may wake up baffled at why they feel exhausted despite getting what seemed like a full night's rest.

In addition to disrupting sleep, PLMD may put a person at risk for some more significant adverse consequences. Studies have shown that the arousals caused by the leg movements are associated with increases in blood pressure and heart rate.

## Treatments for movement disorders

Doctors diagnose RLS and PLMD based on the individual's description of symptoms and, in some cases, observations during an overnight sleep study. Standard neurological examinations often reveal no abnormality.

Several small studies suggest that exercise can ease both RLS and PLMD; walking or other moderate exercise, such as biking or swimming, are good choices. Some people find that cold showers are beneficial, but others prefer heat. Finally, some people with mild RLS may be able to get to sleep by simply massaging their calves or stretching their legs in bed. But most people with moderate to severe RLS need medication.

Drugs that ease the tremors of Parkinson's disease also reduce the number of leg movements and thus improve quality of life for people with RLS and PLMD (see Table 6, page 39). These include levodopa-carbidopa (Sinemet), pramipexole (Mirapex), and

## RLS and PLMD: What's the difference?

| RESTLESS LEGS SYNDROME (RLS) | PERIODIC LIMB MOVEMENT DISORDER (PLMD) |
|---|---|
| Occurs while awake, sometimes preventing sleep. May also cause awakening that makes it difficult to fall asleep again. | Occurs during sleep, causing partial arousals that disrupt sleep. |
| Involves voluntary movements while awake—pacing, knee bends, rocking, or stretching—performed to relieve uncomfortable sensations in the lower legs and knees. Often worse after periods of inactivity and at bedtime. | Involves involuntary movements while asleep, usually repetitive flexing of the big toe, ankle, knee, and hip, typically occurring every 20 to 40 seconds. Episodes last anywhere from a few minutes to several hours. |
| People with RLS are aware of their symptoms, which include aching, burning, tingling, and "creepy-crawly" sensations in the legs. | Affected people usually aren't aware of their symptoms unless a bed partner complains. |
| Diagnosis is based on a person's description of symptoms. | Diagnosis usually requires a sleep study. |

## Table 6: Medications for movement disorders

| GENERIC NAME (BRAND NAME) | SIDE EFFECTS | COMMENTS |
|---|---|---|
| **Benzodiazepines** | | |
| clonazepam (Klonopin)<br>temazepam (Restoril) | Clumsiness or unsteadiness, dizziness, lightheadedness, daytime drowsiness, headache | Should be used with caution by people with sleep apnea or other breathing difficulties; not to be used with alcohol or other depressants; habit-forming; withdrawal symptoms may occur if stopped abruptly. |
| **Dopamine agents** | | |
| levodopa-carbidopa (Sinemet)<br>pramipexole* (Mirapex)<br>ropinirole* (Requip)<br>rotigotine* (Neupro transdermal patch) | Abnormal movements, depression, mental changes, nausea, dizziness | Certain drugs in this class should not be used by people who are sensitive to ergot drugs, who have high blood pressure, who take monoamine oxidase inhibitors (MAOIs), or who have glaucoma. The Neupro patch may cause rash, redness, swelling, or itching. |
| **Opiates** | | |
| oxycodone (OxyContin)<br>oxycodone with acetaminophen (Percocet) | Depressed breathing and circulation, dizziness or lightheadedness, next-day sedation, constipation, nausea, vomiting | Risk of addiction; not to be used by people with sleep apnea; should not be used with alcohol or other depressants. |
| **Anticonvulsants** | | |
| gabapentin (Neurontin)<br>gabapentin enacarbil* (Horizant)<br>pregabalin (Lyrica)<br>valproic acid (Depakene) | Unsteadiness, vision problems, body aches, congestion | Drugs in this class may cause daytime drowsiness. |

*Pramipexole, ropinirole, the rigotine patch, and gabapentin enacarbil are FDA-approved to treat RLS. Other medications in this chart are not approved to treat RLS or PLMD, but physicians have found that they can help people with these conditions.*

ropinirole (Requip). Although the drugs used to treat RLS and PLMD are the same as those used in treating Parkinson's disease, people with these sleep disorders are no more likely to develop Parkinson's disease than other individuals. The FDA has also approved rotigotine (Neupro), a skin patch that delivers a long-acting, once-daily dose of medication to ease restless legs syndrome. Unlike the pills, the medication doesn't go through your digestive system, so you don't have to schedule the drug around meals.

People with mild movement disorders may be prescribed clonazepam (Klonopin) or temazepam (Restoril), which may help them stay asleep during leg movements. Most people who take these medications for insomnia develop a tolerance to them after a few weeks, but this doesn't seem to happen when such drugs are taken for RLS. Antiseizure medications such as gabapentin (Neurontin), which are used to treat epilepsy, are also prescribed for RLS. A related medication called Horizant contains gabapentin enacarbil, a long-acting version of gabapentin. Opiates (opium-

derived drugs) such as oxycodone (OxyContin) may be used to treat people with severe RLS symptoms who don't respond to other treatments. Opiates decrease the discomfort of RLS and, for some, dramatically reduce leg movements at night. But because of the potential for addiction, most physicians are reluctant to treat sleep disturbances with these drugs. However, when properly used, they may provide long-term benefit with little risk of addiction.

# Parasomnias

Parasomnias are strange behaviors that some people engage in during sleep. People with parasomnias may wake up enough to carry out complex actions, but not enough to realize what they are doing. These sleep-disrupting phenomena include sleepwalking, sleep eating, REM sleep behavior disorder, and sleep terrors.

### Somnambulism and somniloquy

Somnambulism, or sleepwalking, occurs during partial awakening from deep sleep. The person's eyes are open but have a confused, glassy appearance. Sometimes sleepwalkers do strange things, such as urinate in a trash can or move furniture. Or they may simply pace or perform repetitive behaviors, such as getting dressed and undressed multiple times. They can be difficult to awaken and typically have no memory of the episode in the morning. There have been reports of somnambulists committing murder, although this is extremely rare. Episodes of sleepwalking are usually brief and benign, with few people endangering themselves or others. Scientists used to believe that sleepwalkers were acting out their dreams, but experts have determined that sleepwalking does not occur during dreaming.

Sleepwalking is common in children, probably because their brains have not yet mastered regulation of sleep and waking. One study found that the incidence of sleepwalking peaks around age 10, affecting about 13% of children at that age. The tendency seems to be inherited. That same study found that among children with sleep terrors (see page 41), which peak around 18 months of age, one-third developed sleepwalking later in childhood, suggesting a possible shared cause. Both conditions were more common among kids whose parents had a history of these sleep disorders.

Although people are more likely to sleepwalk when they're anxious or fatigued, there is little correlation between somnambulism and psychological problems. If the condition continues beyond puberty, the individual should be evaluated to determine whether sleepwalking is the result of nighttime epilepsy or a reaction to medication, extreme stress, or another sleep disorder. If the condition presents a risk of injury, a doctor may prescribe medications such as benzodiazepines.

Somniloquy, or talking in one's sleep, is nothing to worry about. People are more likely to talk in their sleep during times of stress or illness. Talking can occur during any or all stages of sleep. When awakened, people who talk in their sleep rarely remember what they said. Only occasionally can someone who talks in his or her sleep hear and respond to what someone else says.

## Nocturnal eating disorders

There are two distinct nighttime eating disorders.

**Nocturnal eating syndrome** occurs most commonly in people with daytime eating disorders or depression. They are usually light sleepers and wake frequently. Within minutes after getting out of bed, people with this condition raid the refrigerator and begin wolfing down food. Although they aren't really hungry, they can't go back to sleep without eating. In some people with this disorder, overeating occurs only during sleep hours, not during the daytime. The person is awake and fully alert during the episode and can recall it the next day. Nocturnal eating syndrome should be treated as an eating disorder.

**Sleep-related eating disorder** is a combination of a sleep disorder and an eating disorder. People with this disorder experience partial arousals similar to sleepwalking, but respond by eating. Often they consume unhealthful, high-calorie food, such as cookie dough. They report being half-awake or asleep during the episodes and have a very poor memory of the events or no recollection at all. Sleep-related eating disorder occurs more frequently in people with eating disorders and depression. Treatment should address both the sleep disorder and the eating disorder.

Sleep-related eating disorder occurs in children and adults and sometimes can be traced to an illness or traumatic event. A medical evaluation may reveal an ulcer, a history of strict dieting, bulimia, or a sleep problem such as narcolepsy, sleepwalking, sleep apnea, or periodic limb movement disorder. Sometimes medications prescribed for depression or insomnia can cause this disorder. A number of medicines

Two nocturnal eating disorders can cause a person to consume extra food during hours when he or she should be sleeping.

have been tried to treat these disorders, including dopaminergic agents, anticonvulsants, antidepressants, and opiates, but results have been mixed.

## Bedwetting

Bedwetting, known medically as sleep enuresis, is common among young children. It occurs in only a very small percentage of adults. When it does, it is often due to an underlying medical problem or excessive caffeine or beer consumption. In men, an enlarged prostate gland that presses against the bladder may be to blame. Bedwetting may be a side effect of diuretic pills or a sign of diabetes, a bladder or kidney problem, epilepsy, or serious obstructive sleep apnea. Treatment for adult bedwetting depends on the cause.

## REM sleep behavior disorder

Most people make subtle twitching movements during REM sleep, but occasionally sleepers shout, punch, or otherwise act out their dreams. This phenomenon—known as REM sleep behavior disorder—was identified in the 1980s. It's estimated to occur in one in 200 people (0.5%), and nine out of 10 people who have it are men. The disorder nearly always arises after age 50, but there are occasional reports of it occurring in younger adults and children. Approximately 70% of people with REM sleep behavior disorder go on to develop Parkinson's disease, suggesting that similar brain structures are involved in both conditions.

If the person is at risk of harming himself (or herself) or others or is having daytime sleepiness from the sleep disruption, a medium-acting benzodiazepine may help suppress symptoms. Until the problem is under control, people can protect themselves and loved ones by sleeping in a separate room and putting sharp or breakable objects out of reach.

## Nightmares, sleep terrors, and panic attacks

Nightmares, sleep terrors, and sleep-related panic attacks can interrupt sleep.

**Nightmares.** Nightmares, which usually occur in the second half of the sleep period, are bad dreams that become so threatening that a person wakes in a state of fear and agitation. Nightmares occur mainly during REM sleep, when the body barely moves.

Nightmares can be a side effect of certain medications, such as antidepressants, narcotics, cholesterol-lowering statins, and barbiturates. Nightmares can also occur when a person stops taking drugs that temporarily reduce REM sleep, such as benzodiazepines. Alcoholics who stop drinking often experience dream disturbances and nightmares.

If you experience frequent nightmares that aren't linked to medication or substance use, counseling may help. The most common approach is a type of behavioral therapy known as desensitization, in which the sufferer recalls the details of the nightmare and uses relaxation techniques to overcome fear.

**Sleep terrors.** A sleep terror can be quite dramatic to witness. The sleeper might let out a blood-curdling scream, sit bolt upright, and attempt to fight or flee. During an episode, which may last as long as 15 minutes, a person may seem confused and agitated. After the spell is over, he or she is likely to go right back to sleep and later may not remember what happened. For that reason, the episodes are usually more frightening to the parent or other observer than the person having the night terror. It is best to wait for the episode to resolve rather than trying to intervene or wake the sleeper. Make sure the person is safe and not likely to hurt himself or herself by moving about.

Unlike nightmares, sleep terrors occur during non-REM sleep, usually in the first hour or so after going to bed. They appear to run in families and occur most often in children. Up to 6% of children have sleep terrors, which usually occur in the first few years of life and often disappear by early adolescence. Adults with sleep terrors tend to be more agitated, anxious, and aggressive than children who have this problem. When the episodes involve violent or injurious behavior, medical treatment may be recommended. Some doctors prescribe medications such as benzodiazepines that suppress deep sleep. Hypnosis or a relaxation technique known as guided imagery may also be helpful.

**Sleep-related panic attacks.** People may awaken suddenly because of episodes of intense panic characterized by a racing heartbeat, sweating, trembling, breathlessness, or the feeling that they may be dying. Anti-anxiety drugs are often useful for these attacks. ♥

# Narcolepsy

Narcolepsy is a disorder affecting the regulation of the sleep/wake cycle. People with narcolepsy experience bouts of extreme daytime sleepiness and tend to fall asleep suddenly at inappropriate times. These "sleep attacks" seem to arise from an abrupt switch from wakefulness into REM sleep. The brain somehow skips the normal progression of sleep stages, entering into a dreamlike state immediately after a person lies down to sleep—or in the middle of daytime activities, such as talking, eating, or driving. Sudden muscle weakness (known medically as cataplexy) may also occur, causing a person to suddenly go limp or to fall.

The disorder affects about one in 2,000 people and usually appears between ages 15 and 30. It affects men and women equally and has a genetic component: having a close relative makes a person 20 to 40 times more likely to have it. On average, it takes five years of symptoms and visits to five physicians before a diagnosis of narcolepsy is made. This is because sleepiness may be the only symptom. If cataplexy occurs, it may be misdiagnosed as epilepsy or fainting.

In the late 1990s, researchers discovered that many cases of narcolepsy result from the lack of a brain chemical called hypocretin (also called orexin) that normally maintains wakefulness and helps regulate sleep. People with narcolepsy lose the cells that make hypocretin. The discovery of the gene that makes hypocretin and the location of its production in the brain has spurred research into new ways to diagnose and treat this disorder. Researchers have also found a link between narcolepsy and variations in a gene that controls immune function. They speculated that the loss of hypocretin-producing cells may stem from an autoimmune process, in which the body attacks itself.

## Symptoms of narcolepsy

All people with narcolepsy are excessively sleepy and struggle to stay awake during the day, which often

People with narcolepsy frequently experience "sleep attacks," during which they fall asleep at inappropriate times—even while carrying on conversations. They often have trouble completing tasks.

causes them to have great trouble completing tasks. In addition, they may have a number of other symptoms, most of which are manifestations of the REM sleep stage occurring during wakefulness. Most people have more than one but only rarely have all of the following additional symptoms.

**Sleep attacks.** A person may suddenly fall asleep for a few seconds to several minutes when relaxing or even while carrying on a conversation. These attacks may be more frequent when a person is doing something monotonous or repetitive. If REM sleep and dreaming occur immediately, the person sometimes makes conversation that is appropriate to the dream instead of the actual situation.

**Cataplexy.** A person may suddenly lose muscle tone while awake, causing the head to fall forward and the knees to buckle. Most attacks last for less than 30 seconds and may go unnoticed, but in severe cases, the person may fall and stay paralyzed for as long as several minutes. Laughter, anger, or other strong emotions often trigger cataplexy, which occurs when the

## Table 7: Medications for narcolepsy

| GENERIC NAME (BRAND NAME) | USE | SIDE EFFECTS, COMMENTS |
|---|---|---|
| **Stimulants** | | |
| dextroamphetamine (Dexedrine, Adderall)<br><br>methylphenidate (Ritalin, Metadate, Concerta, others) | To counter daytime sleepiness | Nervousness, insomnia, loss of appetite, nausea, dizziness, irregular heartbeat, headaches, changes in blood pressure and pulse, weight loss. Potential for abuse. Should not be used by people who take monoamine oxidase inhibitors (MAOIs) or who have glaucoma. |
| armodafinil* (Nuvigil)<br>modafinil* (Provigil) | To counter daytime sleepiness | Anxiety, headache, nausea, nervousness, insomnia. Less potential for abuse than other stimulants. |
| **Tricyclic antidepressants** | | |
| clomipramine (Anafranil)<br>desipramine (Norpramin)<br>imipramine (Tofranil)<br>protriptyline (Vivactil) | To prevent cataplexy and other REM-related symptoms | Dizziness, dry mouth, blurred vision, weight gain, constipation, trouble urinating, drowsiness, disturbance of heart rhythm. Should not be used with MAOIs or during immediate recovery from heart attack. |
| **SSRI antidepressants** | | |
| fluoxetine (Prozac)<br>paroxetine (Paxil)<br>sertraline (Zoloft)<br>venlafaxine (Effexor) | To prevent cataplexy and other REM-related symptoms | Nausea, dry mouth, headache, loss of appetite, nervousness, diarrhea or constipation, sweating, and sexual problems. Should not be used with MAOIs. |
| **Anticataplectic** | | |
| sodium oxybate* (Xyrem) | To prevent cataplexy, improve nighttime sleep, and reduce daytime sleepiness | Abdominal pain, chills, dizziness, abnormal dreams, drowsiness, stomach discomfort. Must be taken at bedtime and again during the middle of the night. Potential for abuse. |

*Armodafinil, modafinil, and sodium oxybate are FDA-approved to treat narcolepsy symptoms. Other medications in this table are not, but physicians have found they often help people with narcolepsy and therefore prescribe them.*

brain mechanism that paralyzes muscles during REM sleep becomes activated.

**Sleep paralysis.** A terrifying feeling of paralysis may occur during the transition between wakefulness and sleep if the REM stage begins before a person is fully asleep. Although muscle control usually returns within a few minutes, episodes can cause great anxiety.

**Hypnagogic hallucinations.** When REM dreaming occurs during wakefulness, the vivid and often frightening images, known as hypnagogic hallucinations, are difficult to distinguish from reality. A person may see prowlers or believe that his or her house is on fire. This usually happens just at sleep onset or upon awakening. This condition can be confused with mental illness because its symptoms resemble those of some psychotic disorders.

**Disturbed nighttime sleep.** Just as sleep intrudes during the day, unwelcome awakenings can occur at night, depriving people with narcolepsy of restorative rest and worsening their daytime drowsiness. Some feel as if they have hardly slept at all.

**Automatic behavior.** Because of their profound exhaustion, people with narcolepsy perform many routine tasks without being fully aware of what they are doing. For example, one man washed and dried the dishes and then stacked them in the refrigerator, but he had no recollection of doing so.

### Diagnosing narcolepsy

Doctors suspect narcolepsy in people who are excessively sleepy with no other apparent cause, especially if the person also develops one of the other symptoms. Confirming the diagnosis requires an overnight and daytime sleep study. During the overnight study, the person typically falls asleep quickly, goes into REM sleep much faster than usual, and has no other sleep disorder that could cause sleepiness. The next day, the person undergoes a multiple sleep latency test: a series of five nap opportunities, spaced at two-hour intervals throughout the day. A person with narcolepsy falls asleep very quickly and quickly enters REM sleep. Rested people without narcolepsy take longer to fall asleep during the naps or don't sleep at all. If they do sleep, they don't enter REM sleep in the short, 20-minute sleep period permitted during the test.

## Treatments for narcolepsy

Treatment for narcolepsy is geared toward improving wakefulness during the day and preventing REM-related symptoms.

The first-line drugs are two "wakefulness-promoting agents," modafinil (Provigil) and armodafinil (Nuvigil), which are taken once a day in the morning. Exactly how these medications work isn't clear, but they appear to boost levels of the neurotransmitter dopamine. Older drugs, including methylphenidate (Ritalin) or dextroamphetamine (Dexedrine), are less commonly prescribed because of their side effects, which include high blood pressure, extreme weight loss, and addiction (see Table 7, page 43). Even with medications, however, people are never as alert as they would be if they didn't have narcolepsy.

In most people, antidepressants that suppress REM sleep—such as fluoxetine (Prozac), sertraline (Zoloft), paroxetine (Paxil), clomipramine (Anafranil), or venlafaxine (Effexor)—can also prevent cataplexy and other REM-related symptoms.

Another medication for cataplexy is sodium oxybate (Xyrem), also known as gamma hydroxybutyrate (GHB). This medication helps decrease the number of cataplexy episodes and may improve nighttime sleep and reduce daytime sleepiness as well. Because of its chemical properties, it must be taken at bedtime and again during the middle of the night. Xyrem is tightly regulated because of its potential for misuse; it has been associated with criminal acts such as date rape. A new drug called pitolisant (Wakix), which works by enhancing the activity of histamine-producing neurons, also helps keep people awake and prevents cataplexy. In the United States, it is currently available only in clinical trials. ◗

# Disturbances of sleep timing

If your internal clock is out of sync with the usual day/night, wake/sleep pattern, you may long for sleep when you need to be awake—or stay up until the wee hours of the morning without feeling tired. Sleep experts are now beginning to realize that perhaps as many as a quarter of people diagnosed with insomnia may actually have a circadian rhythm disorder. Although this is an area of active research, the diagnosis and treatment of such cases is still in its infancy. This chapter explains various biological clock disturbances and how to best address them.

## Delayed sleep-wake phase disorder

Almost everyone is programmed for a day that lasts slightly longer than 24 hours, but light and other cues keep their sleep/wake cycles in sync with the usual 24-hour schedule. By contrast, "night owls" are less sensitive to these cues. Left to their own devices, they would generally go to sleep and wake up much later than other people each day. Only by relying on external strategies and devices, such as alarm clocks, do they manage to stay in sync with a more conventional schedule. Night owls typically have trouble getting much done in the morning.

If you're a night owl, you may be able to synchronize your schedule with others by going to bed and getting up at the same time every day. However, it's easy for your sleep patterns to go awry when you go on vacation or retire. Night owls often find that a minor shift in sleep/wake cycles—such as the onset of daylight savings time, a coast-to-coast trip, or a weekend of late-night parties—can throw them off kilter unless they force themselves to stick to a schedule.

### Resetting your internal clock

Exposure to bright light as directed by a sleep specialist—a technique known as light therapy—may be useful in treating delayed sleep-wake phase disorder. Upon awakening, you typically sit for 30 minutes facing a specially manufactured box that emits bright light with a minimal amount of ultraviolet light. Initial studies used white light, which contains the entire spectrum of light wavelengths. Later studies have suggested that blue light is the most potent part of the spectrum for resetting the circadian clock.

Another option is to move your bedtime progressively later until you've shifted around the clock and are back in sync. To do this, go to bed three hours later each night. Once you have synchronized your schedule to match that of the other people around you, wake yourself up at the same time each day.

Yet another option for treating delayed sleep-wake phase disorder is to take 0.5 to 3 milligrams of melatonin one hour before your desired bedtime. It also helps to adjust your visual cues even earlier: two hours before bedtime, dim the lights and wear blue light–blocking glasses.

## Advanced sleep-wake phase disorder

People whose body rhythm cycles are shifted much earlier go to bed earlier, wake up in the early morning, and eventually can't stay awake past early evening. This condition is more common among older people. Treatments being studied include bright light therapy in the evening, which helps reset the body's clock, and carefully timed doses of melatonin taken after awakening. Consult a sleep specialist for advice on these measures.

## Non-24-hour sleep-wake rhythm disorder

This unusual circadian rhythm disorder is marked by the continual shifting of the circadian sleep phase later each day, so that people get sleepy at different times each day. This problem is most commonly seen in blind individuals who are not sensitive to the "clock-setting" effects of light. This can be a debilitating condition for some people, creating problems with maintaining a job or desired social life because of the continual mismatch of schedules and internal rhythms. A new melatonin-receptor agonist, tasimelteon (Hetlioz), has been approved for use in blind individuals with this condition.

## Jet lag

Many people find that crossing several time zones makes their internal clocks go haywire. In addition to having headaches, stomach upset, and difficulty concentrating, they may suffer from fitful sleep.

Younger people usually adapt more quickly to time changes than older people. In general, it takes about a day to adjust for every time zone crossed. Most people have more difficulty traveling eastward, but older people may have more symptoms traveling westward.

The standard way to handle jet lag is to shift to the sleep schedule in the new location upon arrival and avoid sleeping at other times, although it may be difficult the first few days. You can also gradually adjust your sleep time prior to leaving (see Figure 7, below). This way your body can start adjusting to the new time zone as soon as possible. Short-term use of timed doses of melatonin or ramelteon to shift circadian rhythms or over-the-counter or prescription sleep aids to help you sleep at night also can be helpful.

---

### Ways to avoid jet lag

There are two basic strategies for minimizing jet lag symptoms. The first—which works best for brief trips just one or two time zones away—is to continue to wake up, eat, and sleep on home time. Schedule appointments for times when you would be alert at home.

On longer trips, try the following measures to help you adjust to the new time zone.

- **Gradually switch before the trip.** For several days before you leave, move mealtimes and bedtime incrementally closer to the schedule of your destination (see Figure 7, at right). Even a partial switch may help.

- **During the flight, drink plenty of fluids, but not caffeine or alcohol.** Caffeine and alcohol promote dehydration, which worsens the symptoms of jet lag. They can also disturb sleep.

- **Switch your bedtime as rapidly as possible upon arrival.** Don't turn in until it's bedtime in the new time zone.

- **Use the sun to help you readjust.** If you need to wake up earlier in the new setting (you've flown west to east), get out in the early morning sun. If you need to wake up later (you've flown east to west), expose yourself to late afternoon sunlight.

### Figure 7: Reset your biological clock

To help reset your biological clock when you're planning a trip through several time zones, as when flying coast to coast, gradually adjust your sleep time before you leave. For example, three days before you plan to travel from the West Coast to the East Coast, go to bed half an hour earlier than usual, and get up half an hour earlier the next morning. The next night, go to bed an hour earlier than usual and get up an hour earlier. The day before you travel, make it 90 minutes. By the fourth day—the day of your trip—you'll find it easier to adjust to your new time zone.

## Sunday insomnia

Some people have trouble falling asleep on Sunday nights. Anxiety about work or school on Monday may play a role, but often, the most important factor is weekend changes in sleep habits. When you stay up late Friday night and sleep in Saturday morning, you are primed to stay up even later Saturday night and sleep in the next day. By Sunday evening, your body's clock is programmed to stay up late, so it's hard to get to sleep on time. People with Sunday insomnia may feel their anxiety mount as they anticipate a difficult night ahead.

The best way to avoid this Sunday insomnia is to maintain the same wake-up time and bedtime on the weekends as during weekdays. If this isn't possible and you end up staying up later than usual on Friday and Saturday, the next best thing is to force yourself to get up at your weekday wake-up time and take an early afternoon nap on Saturday and Sunday. This way, you maintain the same wake-up time but still compensate for your sleep deprivation.

## Shift work

More than 20% of American workers—including health care workers, police officers, security guards, and transit workers—are on the evening or night shift. About 60% to 70% of shift workers experience sleep disturbances. These people fall asleep on the job two to five times more often than day-shift workers do. Sleepiness can be catastrophic for people in these vital roles. Sleep-deprived physicians, for example, make a greater number of errors than their better-rested colleagues. Fatigue often plays a role in overnight rail, plane, truck, and maritime accidents.

Shift workers' sleep disruption can be eased somewhat by incorporating scheduled nap breaks, by rotating shifts from day to evening to night rather than the other way around, or by maintaining the same schedule seven days a week. Shift workers can also benefit from practicing good sleep hygiene (see "Practical tips for sounder sleep," page 13). Dark curtains or eyeshades can keep daylight out, and running a fan can help block external noise.

Shift workers need to enlist the help of family members to get enough sleep while maintaining a schedule at odds with the rest of the world. The most successful shift workers are those who block out time for sleep in advance and then are vigilant about protecting their sleep time from outside intrusions. Light therapy is sometimes recommended to help people get used to a new schedule, as is the short-term use of sleep medications.

## Seasonal affective disorder

In most of North America, winter means less exposure to sunlight. As the days get shorter, some people find themselves depressed, sleepy, and drawn to high-carbohydrate foods.

Researchers speculate that people who suffer from this condition, called seasonal affective disorder (SAD), produce too much melatonin (or are extra-sensitive to normal amounts of this drowsiness-inducing hormone) and don't make enough serotonin, which may encourage carbohydrate cravings. Using a light box that emits bright light for 30 minutes may alleviate the symptoms of SAD and help people wake up in the mornings. Antidepressants can also be helpful. ♥

# Evaluation of sleep disturbances

Surveys suggest that although two-thirds of Americans have sleep problems at some time in their lives, most of them suffer in silence. They enjoy life less, are less productive, and endure more illnesses and accidents at home, on the job, and on the road.

## When to seek help

The American Academy of Sleep Medicine recommends seeking medical advice if sleep deprivation has compromised your daytime functioning for more than a month. Don't hesitate to ask for help when you're sleeping badly following a death in the family or other stressful event. A physician may suggest the short-term use of a sedative to help you sleep at night. This may help you cope better during the day and prevent the development of a long-term sleep disorder.

It's not always easy for people to get an evaluation and treatment for a sleep problem. Doctors trained in the United States receive roughly three hours of instruction on this topic during four years of medical school. According to a National Sleep Foundation survey, most primary care physicians do not routinely ask their patients about sleep. And while most of the physicians who took part in the survey admitted they had limited knowledge about sleep-related matters, more than half did not consult with an expert in sleep medicine. So it's in your best interest to ask your primary care provider for a referral to a sleep specialist.

### Your sleep history

A sleep disturbance cannot be accurately diagnosed unless your physician is familiar with your sleep habits and history. This information may be gleaned from an interview or from written questionnaires that you review and discuss with your doctor (see "A sample sleep history questionnaire," page 51, and "The STOPBANG test for sleep apnea," page 32). Your partner may be able to help answer some of these questions and should contribute to the discussion.

Some people are so used to sleep deprivation that they don't realize they're tired; instead, they may see themselves as lazy, lethargic, or not very motivated. Or they may not think it is unusual to fall asleep at a movie or while sitting at dinner with friends. Someone considered by family members to be a "good napper," able to drop off quickly and sleep through anything, may actually be displaying signs of abnormal sleepiness. Your physician may ask how likely you are to doze off in certain situations. The less appropriate the circumstances (such as waiting in traffic or having a conversation), the more dangerously sleepy you are considered to be (see "How sleepy are you?" below).

---

### How sleepy are you?

Sleep specialists often use this measure, called the Epworth Sleepiness Scale, to gauge a person's level of daytime sleepiness.

Imagine yourself in the following situations, and then select your likelihood of dozing using the 0–3 scale below. Add up these numbers. If you score 11 points or more, consider seeing a physician for an evaluation.

**Scale:** 0 = would never doze
1 = slight chance of dozing
2 = moderate chance of dozing
3 = high chance of dozing

| SITUATION | SCORE |
|---|---|
| Sitting and reading | |
| Watching TV | |
| Sitting inactive in a public place, like a theater or meeting | |
| As a passenger in a car for an hour without a break | |
| Lying down to rest in the afternoon | |
| Sitting and talking to someone | |
| Sitting quietly after lunch (when you've had no alcohol) | |
| In a car while stopped in traffic | |
| TOTAL | |

---

### The psychiatric interview

Sleep disturbances, particularly insomnia, are often related to psychological difficulties that respond well to treatment once they've been identified. Physicians may screen problem sleepers for symptoms of depression, anxiety, childhood physical or sexual abuse, or other psychological problems or traumatic experiences. If one of these conditions is diagnosed, your primary care physician may refer you to a psychologist or psychiatrist for treatment.

## Sleep testing

Most people with sleep problems don't need to visit a sleep laboratory. Insomnia and circadian rhythm disorders, for example, can be diagnosed in the doctor's office based on a thorough history and physical examination. However, when a doctor suspects a sleep disorder such as narcolepsy, periodic limb movement disorder, sleep apnea, or one of the parasomnias, he or she may recommend formal sleep testing, which can be done in a sleep laboratory or with portable devices you can use at home.

Fees depend on the level of testing required. Some people require a one-time consultation with a sleep specialist, which may run a few hundred dollars. Staying overnight in a sleep laboratory costs between $800 and $1,500. Home tests can cost from $300 to $600. Check with your insurance company in advance because reimbursement varies and may depend on your diagnosis.

The American Academy of Sleep Medicine has a listing of more than 2,500 accredited sleep disorders centers and more than 5,600 board-certified sleep specialists (see "Resources," page 52). Some centers allow you to make an appointment directly, while others require a physician referral. The center will request medical records and may send you a sleep questionnaire or diary to use before your visit. You may also be asked to change your sleep habits in certain ways before scheduling the visit. Sometimes these changes alone correct the problem.

### Laboratory sleep tests

These tests provide the most reliable way of diagnosing sleep fragmentation disorders such as obstructive sleep apnea, periodic limb movement disorder, or seizure disorders and determining their severity. When you spend the night in a sleep laboratory, you'll wear your own nightclothes and you can use a pillow from home. You can take your regular medications, but the clinicians will need to know what they are. The lab usually provides a regular bed in a private room. After a technician sets up the sleep-monitoring equipment, you'll be left alone to relax until bedtime. Throughout the night, laboratory staff will monitor the instruments in a nearby control room.

Procedures used may include the following.

**Polysomnography.** In this procedure, small wafer-thin electrodes and other sensors are pasted on specific body sites to take a variety of readings during the night. They may be placed on your scalp to track brain waves; under your chin to measure fluctuations in muscle tension (called an electromyogram, or EMG); near your eyes to measure eye movements; near your nostrils to measure airflow; on your earlobe or finger to measure the amount of oxygen in your blood (using a device called an oximeter); on your chest or back to record heart rate and rhythm; on your legs to record twitches or jerks; and over your rib muscles or around the rib cage and abdomen to monitor breathing.

Readings are collected on a single printout (called a polysomnogram) and analyzed by a technician and physician. If a breathing problem is detected early on, you may be awakened and given treatment, such as PAP, during the second half of the night. This allows the sleep experts to monitor how well the treatment works for you. Sometimes this process requires two nights. If your doctor suspects that you have a seizure disorder, you may also undergo a full electroencephalogram (EEG) during the night.

**Audio and video recording.** Audio equipment may be used to record snoring, talking during sleep, or other sounds. A video may also be taken to compare with the polysomnogram. This may show, for example, that you snore only when in a certain position. Signs of movement disorders (such as periodic limb movement disorder) or parasomnias will probably be apparent on the video.

**Daytime sleep tests.** After a night in the sleep lab, your doctor may want you to take one or more daytime sleep tests as well.

One, called the multiple sleep latency test, measures how long it takes you to drift off while lying down in a quiet room and also determines what stages of sleep you experience during a brief nap. The procedure is usually repeated four or five times during the day at two-hour intervals. This test assesses how sleepy you are and looks for signs of narcolepsy. Falling asleep within eight minutes each time indicates extreme sleepiness. A person who enters REM sleep very quickly (within about 20 minutes) likely has narcolepsy.

In a less common test, called the maintenance of wakefulness test, you're given the opposite instructions: try to stay awake. This ability is also affected by the degree of sleepiness. People are sometimes given both tests at different times. The Federal Aviation Association uses this test to ensure that pilots treated for sleep apnea are sufficiently awake and alert to fly.

### Home-based tests

For people who, based on their symptoms, probably have moderate to severe obstructive sleep apnea and who have no other significant medical problems, home sleep monitoring may be almost as effective as a night in the sleep lab. Portable home recording devices also may be used when polysomnography is not available and a person's symptoms suggest a need for immediate treatment or when a person is bedridden or medically unstable and cannot be moved. Finally, home-based tests can provide an easy way for a physician to evaluate the effectiveness of a treatment.

The big advantage of a home sleep test is its convenience. You sleep in your own bed, not an unfamiliar hospital bed, and you do the test based on your schedule, not when a sleep center can fit you in. But there are disadvantages, too. There's no technician around to reattach a sensor or wire if it comes loose, so you must repeat the test if this happens. In addition, home monitors detect only OSA, not other sleep disorders, which means that some people still end up needing a full sleep lab test. And because home-based tests are not as sensitive, they may understate the severity of OSA or miss mild sleep apnea altogether.

**Apnea detectors.** Portable detection kits come in many makes and models. There are simple ones that measure only the amount of oxygen in the blood-stream. Most also monitor other breathing variables—air flow, chest movement (to detect breathing patterns), and heart rate or the heart's electrical activity. Some portable devices can also detect snoring or leg movement. Very few measure brain activity and stages of sleep, information that is needed to identify other types of sleep disorders.

Once you have the kit, you attach the various sensors to your body before going to bed: a clip on your fingertip tracks your heart rate and the amount of oxygen in the bloodstream; a sensor that loops over the ears and sits below the nose monitors airflow and snoring; an elastic band around the chest records breathing patterns. With everything in place, you go to sleep in your own bed. The information is stored on a data card that your doctor downloads and interprets.

**Wrist actigraphy.** A wristwatch-sized monitoring device that automatically records arm or leg movements can be used to track periods of sleep and wakefulness at night. Although it cannot determine the stage of sleep, it can help clarify ambiguous aspects of a sleep diary—such as entries reporting long hours of sleep but exhaustion the next day—or assess the effectiveness of medical treatment. The actigraphy device may reveal that brief awakenings during the night are unknowingly disturbing sleep. In some studies, wrist actigraphy was almost 90% accurate in determining whether a person was asleep. This type of monitoring is now included in many wearable fitness devices and smart watches.

## Looking forward to a healthier future

This report has focused on the ways sleep disturbances can harm your health, but it's worth taking a moment to look at the flip side—the benefits of routinely getting a good night's rest. The encouraging news is that if you successfully conquer your sleep problems, you will not only have more refreshing sleep at night, but also better energy, productivity, and mental well-being during the day. After a few weeks of healthy sleep, some people report feeling like a "whole new person." While there are no guarantees that you can always get eight hours of uninterrupted rest, with proper treatment, you can reasonably expect improvements in your sleep—and your overall quality of life. ▼

# A sample sleep history questionnaire

*Your physician may ask you some of the following questions during an evaluation for a sleep problem. You may find it helpful to write down your answers to these questions and bring the completed questionnaire to the exam so you and your doctor can discuss it.*

What bothers you most about your sleep?

_____

_____

How long have you had trouble sleeping, and what do you think started the problem? Did it come on suddenly?

_____

_____

How would you describe your usual night's sleep?

_____

_____

What time do you go to bed, and when do you wake up?

_____

_____

How long does it take you to fall asleep?

_____

Once you're asleep, do you sleep through the night or wake up frequently?

_____

_____

What's your bedroom like?

_____

_____

What do you do in the few hours before bedtime?

_____

_____

Do you follow the same sleep pattern during the week and on weekends? If not, how are weekends different?

_____

_____

How well do you sleep on the first few nights when you're away from home? At home, do you sleep better in your bedroom or in another room in the house?

_____

_____

Do you often feel sleepy during the day?

_____

Do you fall asleep at inappropriate times or places?

_____

Do allergies or nasal congestion bother you at night?

_____

_____

Have you ever been in a car accident or had a close call because you nodded off at the wheel?

_____

_____

Do you have physical aches and pains that interfere with sleep?

_____

_____

What medications or drugs (including alcohol and nicotine) do you use? Have you ever taken sleep medications? If so, which ones?

_____

_____

Do you often have indigestion at night?

_____

Do you ever feel discomfort or a fidgety sensation in your legs and feet when you lie down? Do you have to get up and walk around to relieve the feeling?

_____

_____

Do you kick or thrash around at night?

_____

Do you ever have trouble breathing when you lie down, or do you awaken because it's hard to breathe?

_____

Does your bed partner or roommate mention that you snore loudly or gasp for air at night?

_____

_____

Do you ever awaken with a choking sensation or a sour taste in your mouth?

_____

_____

Do you wake up with a headache or with cramps in your legs?

_____

_____

How have you been feeling emotionally? Does your life seem to be going as well as you would like?

_____

_____

# Resources

## Organizations

**American Academy of Sleep Medicine**
2510 N. Frontage Road
Darien, IL 60561
630-737-9700
www.sleepeducation.org

Dedicated to the advancement of sleep medicine and related research, this organization also maintains the Sleep Education website to provide the public with information on sleep disorders as well as contact information for accredited sleep centers.

**American Sleep Apnea Association**
641 S St. NW, 3rd Floor
Washington, DC 20001
888-293-3650 (toll-free)
www.sleepapnea.org

This nonprofit organization provides information on sleep apnea via brochures, a newsletter, and videos. It also operates a network of support groups throughout the country.

**Narcolepsy Network**
P.O. Box 2178
Lynnwood, WA 98036
888-292-6522 (toll-free)
www.narcolepsynetwork.org

This organization offers educational materials on narcolepsy, as well as help in finding support groups.

**National Center on Sleep Disorders Research**
National Heart, Lung, and Blood Institute, NIH
6701 Rockledge Drive
Bethesda, MD 20892
www.nhlbi.nih.gov/about/org/ncsdr

This federal center, part of the National Institutes of Health, coordinates government-supported sleep research, training, and education. It offers a number of free publications about sleep disorders.

**National Sleep Foundation**
1010 N. Glebe Road, Suite 310
Arlington, VA 22201
703-243-1697
www.sleepfoundation.org

This nonprofit foundation helps consumers locate sleep centers and provides information on a variety of sleep topics.

**Restless Legs Syndrome Foundation, Inc.**
3006 Bee Caves Road, Suite D206
Austin, TX 78746
512-366-9109
www.rls.org

This nonprofit foundation distributes brochures and provides information on restless legs syndrome. It also maintains a list of support groups located throughout the country.

## Websites

**CBT-i Coach**
https://mobile.va.gov/app/cbt-i-coach

This free app was developed for military veterans and service members for use with a health care professional. But it can serve as a stand-alone educational tool about CBT-i treatment for civilians as well.

**Conquering Insomnia Program**
www.cbtforinsomnia.com

This cognitive behavioral therapy program, developed at Harvard Medical School and the University of Massachusetts Medical Center, is available for purchase as either an online program or in CD format.

**MyApnea**
https://myapnea.org

MyApnea is a community of patients, doctors, and researchers (including those from three Harvard teaching hospitals) trying to improve the diagnosis and treatment of sleep apnea. It includes an online forum where people with sleep apnea share information about their experiences, including sleep studies, using PAP machines, and other concerns.

**Sleep and Health Education Program**
http://healthysleep.med.harvard.edu

Created by Harvard Medical School's Division of Sleep Medicine and the WGBH Educational Foundation, this site aims to help the general public understand sleep and to get the sleep they need.

**Sleepio**
www.sleepio.com

Created by researchers in the United Kingdom, this online sleep improvement program uses cognitive behavioral therapy to address sleep problems.

**Welltrinsic Sleep Network**
www.welltrinsic.com

This nationwide network of board-certified sleep specialists and accredited sleep centers offers a "Find a Sleep Doctor" feature and sleep wellness program.

## Harvard Special Health Reports

The following Special Health Reports from Harvard Medical School elaborate on topics in this report. To order, call 877-649-9457 (toll-free) or go to www.health.harvard.edu.

**Anxiety and Stress Disorders: A guide to managing panic attacks, phobias, PTSD, OCD, social anxiety disorder, and related conditions**
Theodore Murray, M.D., Medical Editor
(Harvard Medical School, 2018)

Anxiety can be a sleep stealer. This report details ways of coping with multiple types of anxiety disorders, including cognitive behavioral therapy, medication, and relaxation techniques.

**Better Bladder and Bowel Control**
May M. Wakamatsu, M.D., Joseph A. Grocela, M.D., and Liliana Bordeianou, M.D., Medical Editors
(Harvard Medical School, 2017)

An estimated 20 million American adults have urinary incontinence, and 19 million have fecal incontinence. The good news is that treatments are becoming more effective and less